Destination: Fatherhood

by Joe Kelly

GARRICK
STREET
PRESS

Publisher *Mike Sanders*
Executive Managing Editor *Billy Fields*
Senior Acquisitions Editor *Brook Farling*
Development Editor *Kayla Dugger*
Senior Production Editor *Janette Lynn*
Cover Designer *Rebecca Batchelor*
Book Designer *William Thomas*
Indexer *Heather McNeill*
Layout *Brian Massey*
Proofreader *Tricia Liebig*

First published in 2014 in the United States by DK Publishing
6081 E. 82nd Street, Indianapolis, Indiana 46250

001–316088–JAN2019

This 2019 edition is published by Garrick Street Press, an imprint of
Dorling Kindersley Limited

Note: This publication contains the opinions and ideas of its authors. It is
intended to provide helpful and informative material on the subject matter
covered. It is sold with the understanding that the authors and publisher
are not engaged in rendering professional services in the book. If the
reader requires personal assistance or advice, a competent professional
should be consulted. The authors and publisher specifically disclaim any
responsibility for any liability, loss, or risk, personal or otherwise, which is
incurred as a consequence, directly or indirectly, of the use and application
of any of the contents of this book.

ISBN: 978-1-4654-8883-1
Library of Congress Catalog Number: 2018967852

For Maya Philipson, family and friend.

Contents

Part 4: Turning the Corner 185

10   Ready to Launch: Planning for the Big Day 187

11   Delivery Day 199

Introduction

So you're a dad-to-be. Congratulations! I'm convinced that fatherhood is the most remarkable thing that can happen to a man. There's a chance that someone gave you this book as a gift. Maybe you're looking at it now just to be polite. Maybe the person who gave it to you (a woman, perhaps?) is watching to see if you crack it open.

If you're skeptical, I don't blame you. Think about it: most dads through history did their fathering without ever reading a book. However, over the last century or so, boys have rarely been taught about helping a female loved one through pregnancy, taking care of infants, or raising older children. Did your father teach your about morning sickness or burping babies? Probably not—but then, your grandfather probably didn't teach that to your dad, either.

As a result, even in this age of changing attitudes about the roles of men and women, most men have few (if any) road maps for transforming from a "guy who isn't a dad" into that mysterious entity known as "Dad."

So, what is that transformation like? Have you ever been on a roller coaster? Then you have a taste of what it's like to become a dad—excitement, screams, wild laughter, panic, hanging on for the ride, and more. But unlike a roller coaster, which brings you back to the same place you started, fatherhood transports you to new adventures every day. It's also a bit hard to wrap your mind around, especially when you're still expecting.

You are not alone. *Destination: Fatherhood* lays out a clear, simple map for your journey that combines fathering "wisdom of the ages" with new insights to guide you through pregnancy, childbirth, and bringing your beautiful baby home.

In these pages, you'll find how to do the following:

- Stake and keep a central role throughout birthing classes, your partner's doctors' visits, labor, delivery, and the first days of your child's new life.

- Combine your natural instincts and new knowledge to effectively support your partner throughout her pregnancy.

- Embrace and enjoy your new baby and your life as a father.

- Work together with your baby's mother to co-parent this child for years to come.

- Experience the wonder of fatherhood, this amazing new phase in your life as a man.

Fair warning: this book won't help you win a perfect parenting award—but then, no other father (or mother) in history has won one either. But I can promise that you'll come away with a good toolbox that can help you deal with the most common situations and challenges of expectant fatherhood. You'll also start to sense how much you already know about getting ready for—and loving—a brand-new baby.

Through the centuries, millions of dads have swelled with pride and recoiled from uncertainty. Yet somehow, the human species keeps surviving and thriving through the good—if imperfect—parenting of fathers and mothers. So as you step onto the pregnancy ride and enter the ups and downs of fatherhood, keep this book nearby to help you survive and enjoy the thrills of becoming and being a dad.

How This Book Is Organized

I've divided the book into four parts:

Part 1, It's Daddy Time, covers common anxieties and excitement expectant fathers experience and lays out some ideas for creating your own way to be a dad. In this part, I deal with the dynamics and emotions you and your partner will have as the baby's birth draws closer. You also get basic information on how a "normal" pregnancy works and how to get and stay healthy throughout. You then learn about options when faced with fertility issues, such as artificial insemination and adoption. I end this part with a discussion about sex and sexuality during pregnancy.

Part 2, The Pregnancy Path, walks you through the nine months from conception to birth, describing what's happening to the fetus, your partner, and you in each trimester. You learn how to be an effective wingman for your partner by attending childbirth classes and making your last times alone together special. You also get a rundown on some of the twists pregnancy can take, such as health issues for your partner, having multiple babies, and miscarriage.

Part 3, The New Life Plan, covers how to get your life, work, and environment in order for a newborn. In this part, you learn how to choose obstetric, pediatric, and daycare professionals. There's also guidance on the essentials you need in the nursery and the rest of your home before your baby comes home. You even get the low-down on gear to keep the baby safe—and keep you sane—when you leave home. I close with a discussion about preparing your workplace, work life, and finances for the transition to fatherhood.

Part 4, Turning the Corner, shows how to prepare for labor and delivery through birth plans, preparation for the hospital, and ahead-of-time delivery room decisions. You learn the stages of labor and delivery and the details of your job as your partner's birthing partner and coach. You also get a rundown of the basics for bringing your baby home, from holding and feeding to burping and changing diapers. Finally, I discuss ways to share parenting between you and your partner—and help you develop your own fathering vision.

Extras

Look for these handy sidebars throughout the book. They have important information you need to know to get the most out of your entry into fatherhood.

Say, Dad

These sidebars contain humorous, inspirational, and instructive quotes from or about famous and not-so-famous fathers.

Baby Steps

You find simple (and sometimes counter-intuitive) tips you can use to smooth the journey for you, her, and your baby in these sidebars.

 Pregnant Pause

These sidebars give you warnings on the common dangers, missteps, and myths concerning pregnancy and childbirth.

 Attention, Please

In these sidebars, you learn how to watch out for your partner's needs (and your own) as you build deep, life-long family bonds.

A Note About Word Use

When writing about fatherhood, I think it's important to use terms that include every person who is—or is about to be—a parent. For example, good parenting isn't dependent on or determined by whether the parents are (or are not) married, or whether their sexuality is the same as yours or mine. Many fathers aren't married to the mothers of their children, and some children are raised by two dads. Therefore, you will rarely see the words "husband" or "wife" in this book; instead, you'll see the term *partner.*

I readily admit that my "substitute" term seems short on the love, romance, and warmth that flows through vibrant intimate relationships like a good marriage (or a good nonmarriage). On the other hand, strong and lasting relationships—like the 35 years I've spent (so far) with my wife Nancy—are partnerships. In any case, that's the word I use—and if you think of something better, please write me!

Along a similar line, when it comes to discussing babies, I never refer to a child as "it." Instead, you'll see that I alternate the terms *she* and *he* by chapter.

Acknowledgments

Thanks to Will Glennon, Bill Klatte, Armin Brott, Michael Kimmel, Michael Kieschnick, Jackson Katz, Paul Banas, and John Badalament for their guidance and work on fathering and manhood. I'm especially grateful for the medical perspective of Joy Dorscher, MD, associate dean of the University of North Dakota Medical School; Michael Jennis, MD, chief of the neonatal intensive care unit at the Kaiser Oakland (CA) Medical Center; and Leslie Kardos, MD, chief of gynecology at the California Pacific Medical Center and instructor at the University of California-San Francisco Medical School.

For their expert guidance, my gratitude to Bill Trzeciak; Mark Stelzner; Rabbi Naomi Tzril Saks, MDiv, BCC; Mark Nemeth; Ryan Ruffcorn; Mike Moore; R. Clarence Jones; Kenny Bodanis; Emily Doskow; Sam Simmons; Melissa Froehle; Paul Masiarchin; Lyle Wildes; Bill Wilson; Bob Smith, MD; and Judge David W. Peterson, JD. The thousands of men who've shared their stories with me over the years teach me so much and have my respect every day. A very special thanks to the crew at Starbucks store #8912 in Emeryville, California, for hosting me while writing the book.

Material from *The Body Myth: Adult Women and the Pressure to Be Perfect* is adapted and used by permission of the copyright holders, Margo Maine, PhD, and Joe Kelly.

For help in birthing the book, my thanks to Brook Farling, Kayla Dugger, Marilyn Allen, Coleen O'Shea, Ryan Goei, Steve Knauss, Dusty Johnson, the late Kevin Karr, and Mike Sanders.

Most of all, thanks to the people who still keep me on my toes as a dad (and, now, granddad): Mavis Gruver, Nia Kelly, Nancy Gruver, Maya Phlipson, Mark Stelzner, Samuel Elliot Kelly Stelzner, and Lucy and Greta Vokes-Ruffcorn.

Trademarks

It's Daddy Time

You're already on an amazing journey called fatherhood. There's no end of the line on this road; "Destination: Fatherhood" is a state of being present and positive in your child's life now and for years to come.

The more you think about fathering, the more overwhelming it may seem. This part of the book tackles the thrills and turmoil that are normal for expectant dads. It provides perspective on your own parents and ways to start planning how you will parent your child— which could be very similar or very different from the parenting you received. I also show you how to cope with the often-intense relationship and emotional issues you and your partner may face.

In this part, I then give you a review of the male and female reproductive systems and how they're designed to work. I also discuss what happens when the complex fertility process presents you with challenges—along with descriptions of how fertility treatments and other options can help you respond to those challenges.

And because most men wonder whether sex will be challenging (or even possible) during pregnancy, I close this part by telling you about the many ways that sexuality and sexual practices during pregnancy can actually draw you and your partner closer together!

Crossing Over to Father Land

In This Chapter

- Preparing for fatherhood
- Overcoming fears you may have about being a father
- Managing your expectations
- Learning from veteran parents
- Embracing your new role

I became a dad in 1980 and a grandpa in 2012. For the last 22 years, my work has been interviewing fathers and stepfathers, teaching fathering classes, and writing books and articles about fathering.

Here are the two most important things I've learned from all that experience:

1. A millennia-long natural heritage of fathering provides a solid foundation for dads (including you) today.

2. Despite all that collective fathering experience, it still takes conscious effort (and sometimes a bit of pushiness) for a man to stay fully involved in pregnancy, childbirth, and child rearing.

Don't worry if you don't feel entirely ready for the birth of your child—no father is. That's because this baby has never been born before. Plus, knowing everything ahead of time would take a lot of fun out the experience. So don't fight it, accept it!

This chapter gives you some hints on how to prepare yourself for fathering, so you can get from now to delivery day—and beyond!

Being "Prepared" for Fatherhood

I've never met a dad who says he really knew what fatherhood would be like before the baby was born. I've been a dad for more than 30 years and a fathering educator for more than 20 years, and I still haven't found adequate words to describe the transition from "not a dad" to "Dad."

When your baby is born, you'll cross over into this new terrain where your previous preparation will help but only take you so far. You'll go the rest of the way on instinct and love for your unique child.

 Say, Dad

Despite my fears of fatherhood, I had strong nurturing urges. These I sublimated for years with a succession of cats upon whom I doted to a sometimes embarrassing degree.

—Dan Greenburg, author

This transformation can be a bit intimidating to contemplate, but it is simultaneously an incredible adventure. I'm convinced that becoming a father is the most profound experience any man can have. You'll do, say, and feel things you never did, said, or felt before. It will be exhilarating, scary, euphoric, heartbreaking, thrilling, confusing, amazing, proud, and many other sensations, too.

Fortunately, this powerful and fulfilling journey begins even before the moment of birth, as you begin to sense that fatherhood is a blast!

Common Fears and Concerns

If you're like most soon-to-be new dads, you have questions that are hard to talk about with anyone else. Facing this major change on your life, you may feel unsure, afraid, and confused. That's because you've never been a dad before, and it's impossible to know exactly what it'll be like for you. Expectant father questions range from practical to very personal, such as the following:

- Can I share my partner with someone else—even a baby?

- Can I be certain that this is *my* child?

- Will I love (or even like) the baby?

- Will I know how to raise a child?

- Do I really want to go through with this?

- Does fatherhood mean I can't have fun anymore?

- What if my baby daughter grows up and has to deal with teenage boys who act like I did as a kid?

- Do I have or can I make enough money to afford a family?

- Will I break the baby?

- Will I get sick and pass out in the delivery room?

These questions are completely normal. You aren't alone when you wonder, worry, or are uncertain about your partner's pregnancy—and becoming a new dad.

On top of all this unknown territory, you sense (rightly) that a little baby will soon depend on you for his very survival over the next few years. How often has that ever happened to you before? Probably never.

 Pregnant Pause

You will play a crucial role in your child's life, so be a big part of his life from this day forward. By actively involving yourself, you can be a good father—the one your child needs you to be.

Once you're a father, you'll need to protect, support, and guide your child for a long time. Your child is likely to live under your roof for 18 to 20 years, and (if you're lucky) continue seeking your guidance and encouragement for years afterward.

Don't be surprised if that gives you a greater sense of dread than what you commonly experience during the last 30 minutes of a horror movie. Ask the dad next door; he'll confirm that dread can be a recurring feeling for fathers. Of course, just because those sensations are normal doesn't make them pleasant.

However, it does help to know this: you change as a man because you're a father. You may not know how your actions will affect your baby, but they will. Plus, there's no way to know what's going to happen next in your child's life, no matter his age. The important thing is to be involved, responsible, teachable, and willing to give it your all.

Being a father is an obligation. Your child will rely on you, and your parenting has lasting influence—you will be your child's father until the day *your child* dies. However, involved fathers will tell you that being a dad is much more than an obligation. The more engaged you are in your baby's life, the more you'll recognize fatherhood as an opportunity to shape your child into someone who's emotionally healthy and productive.

You should also know that, as an expectant parent, you have the instincts to protect and provide for your new baby. These instincts are very important and versatile, so use them to your and your child's advantage.

For example, make sure you keep a broad and healthy definition of being a provider—one that goes well beyond your important financial and material contributions. Your instincts give you the capacity to supply him with inspiration, time, expectations, affection, knowledge, fun, reassurance, attention, adventure, and so much more.

My daughters are adults now, and I couldn't tell you my weekly pay the year they were born. However, I can tell you in detail about the first time I heard them laugh, or the colic-filled night that I got them to sleep when my wife couldn't. You can't buy memories like these, and that's what it means to be a father who provides.

In other words, full engagement in your child's life matters far more than a full wallet.

Provide your partner and your child with a large and steady dose of your energy, warmth, masculinity, stories, physicality, love of risk, heritage—in other words, all the wonderful things that make up a man and father.

Even though you're new at this, you really can enjoy and excel at being a dad. You can be a great co-parent with your partner, applying your unique talents and experiences to the fabulous challenge of raising another human being.

Somehow fathers, mothers, and babies have survived this process for millennia. You, too, will make it through your moments of panic and euphoria, because you'll be able to draw on abilities you may not know you have.

Will I Love My Baby?

Perhaps the most basic fear for an expectant dad is whether he'll love his baby. We fathers all have moments (sometimes, extended ones) of feeling and thinking all kinds of negative things about fatherhood. That happens both before the child is born and during the exhausting early weeks and months after the birth. As author Michael Lewis writes, "Fatherhood can be demoralizing. I usually wound up the day curled in a little ball of fatigue, drowning in self-pity. … I expected to feel overcome with joy, while instead I often felt only puzzled."

 Baby Steps

Stay connected and involved in raising this precious child, and the loving times will far outnumber the maddening times.

Meanwhile, many other folks may expect us to proclaim how thrilled we are, tempting us to engage in elaborate deceptions. When you worry or get frustrated about the situation, remember the following key points.

* You don't have to hide your frustrations, fears, or ambivalence about becoming a dad. If you share them with a veteran dad—and even with your partner—you'll find you're not alone.

* Frustration, fear, and ambivalence don't prevent love or indicate you don't love your baby. Paradoxically, the nitty-gritty of real life can draw you closer to your child; for example, changing a dirty diaper gives you the chance to look in your baby's eyes, babble at him, and get to know him.

* You will love your baby.

Just as in any other human relationship, you'll probably feel more loving toward your child at certain times than you do at others. Nevertheless, your bond is always there. While he's a child and you're the grown-up, it's your job to nurture and strengthen that bond.

If You Didn't Have a Good Role Model

If your parents were cruel or abusive to you during your childhood, you may fear that you won't be good at fathering, or that you may even continue the cycle of negative behavior. How do know if you were abused? Did a parent, stepparent, or other respected adult ever do the following:

* Punch, slap, kick, or throw you in anger?

* Ridicule you or call you names?

* Perform a sexual act on or with you?

* Use emotional or psychological cruelty to threaten or manipulate you?

* Abuse alcohol or other drugs?

Statistically, adults who were abused as children are more likely to—*although not predestined to*—abuse their own kids or their partner. They're also more likely to accept abuse of their kids or themselves as normal. The generational cycle of abuse is fed by adult survivors' understandable reluctance to confront pain and anger from their own childhood. In other words, the short-term, "triage" defense of denial can morph into an ongoing and dangerous way of life if not dealt with in adulthood.

For example, my father was an alcoholic. Alcoholics do crazy things when they're drinking, and even sometimes when they're not. As a kid, I didn't know anything about alcoholism, so I accepted my father's behavior as normal. I didn't have anything else to compare to, so I assumed the "typical" father behaved like that.

Yet his alcoholism did not make my father a worthless parent. He was a good man and made wonderful contributions to my life. Still, he had a disease that made him do some ugly, harmful things. And it took conscious effort for me as an adult, along with the loving support of friends, to learn that many of my father's behaviors were not normal—or healthy—parenting.

It is absolutely essential for you to take an honest look at any emotional, physical, or sexual abuse you may have survived as a child so you can successfully break the cycle. Verbal, emotional, and physical abuse scar a child, and, over the long haul, it doesn't make the adult feel any better either. So don't do it—don't let a blind eye on your past drag you down into harming your kid.

 Pregnant Pause

You can find resources for yourself from Adult Survivors of Child Abuse (ascasupport.org/resources. php), Adult Survivors of Childhood Sexual Abuse (rainn.org), and Futures Without Violence (future-swithoutviolence.org). These books are also great: *Beginning to Heal: A First Book for Men and Women Who Were Sexually Abused As Children* by Ellen Bass and Laura Davis and *Allies in Healing: When the Person You Love was Sexually Abused as a Child* by Laura Davis.

Most important, be aware of what you must do as a father to your child, now that you're no longer a child yourself. Actively seek and find constructive and nonviolent ways to deal with stress, frustration, exhaustion, fear, and pain, such as the following.

- Go for a walk or to the gym.

- Call or visit a friend for a break in your routine and to talk about what's going on.

- Create a regularly scheduled time for you and your partner to calmly discuss what's happening; think of it as a family meeting, if that helps.

- Take a "time out" to step away from the stress, even if it's just a few minutes of breathing deeply or walking around the backyard.

Don't be afraid to ask for help—even professional help—to get you there. This greatly reduces the chance that you will replay a cycle that would hurt your precious baby.

Even better, you will soon find that breaking the cycle makes it easier to fully experience and enjoy the pride, excitement, affection, joy, and unconditional love your child will bring into your life. Trust me, there's no greater feeling in the world.

Dealing with Jealousy

As your partner progresses in her pregnancy, she'll probably get a lot of attention. People will be asking her questions, sharing stories, offering sympathy, and all the rest. At those times, you may feel left out or in the background.

In addition, because your partner's attention is focused on her own body, how the baby is doing, and the major changes happening now and later when the baby comes, you may feel like you're not getting the attention you're used to—or feel you deserve—from her.

Most expectant dads encounter feelings of jealousy or resentment at some point. When those feelings stir within you, it's essential for you bring them out and talk about them with someone you trust—including your partner.

That can be very hard, because jealously and resentment are powerful emotions that don't always respond quickly to logic and reason.

Plus, you may feel like you don't want (or deserve) to bother her with your problems. However, as fathering expert Armin Brott says, jealousy is a dangerous thing to bury: "Left unspoken, your feelings may make you resent both your wife and your baby and could damage your marriage and your experience of fatherhood."

 Attention, Please

When discussing difficult feelings, try to do it when both of you are calm—not in the middle of a tense or loaded situation. This increases the chance you can hear each other with empathy and love.

To help yourself through these times, check in with your partner regularly. Ask how she's doing. When you demonstrate your caring for her, it's easier to give her the gift of sharing how you're doing and what you're thinking, even if it isn't "logical." Tell her when you're feeling less than enthusiastic about the sleep disruption (when she gets up to pee every half hour), all the looming changes, and being seen as second string on the pregnancy team.

You can also sustain intimacy by continuing to date your partner, even though she's pregnant. Schedule a night or afternoon out together regularly. Make the date its very own special event, rather than an appendage to something you're already doing. (This is a good strategy for after the baby arrives, too.) It doesn't have to be fancy—just be sure you and your partner are alone together. Try talking about something other than pregnancy and parenting. That will strengthen your relationship and remind you both that your lives include other important things.

Today's Dad

You're having a baby at a time in history when there is more freedom and acceptance for "nontraditional" ways of being a father than during previous generations. (I'll talk about some specific choices and options in Chapters 9 and 13.)

First, let's acknowledge that this growing father freedom is both exciting and sometimes terrifying. It's great to have more room to maneuver, and it can be scary to create your own kind of fathering without a ton of readily visible examples to follow.

 Say, Dad

Once, when I was a boy, the world wasn't so big and I could see everywhere. That was when my father was a hero and not a human.

—Markus Zusak, author

What Little Boys Are Made Of

When you think of the role a mother plays in raising a child, terms like *feeding*, *nurturing*, and *comforting* might spring to mind. But what does it mean to "father" a child—more than the actual biological part, I mean?

Our society doesn't invest nearly as much time and attention to preparing boys to become fathers as it does preparing girls to become mothers. And we as a society need to start requiring boys to learn about and practice the task of being fathers.

To illustrate, let's look at two esteemed organizations dedicated to developing kids into well-rounded adults: the Boy Scouts of America (BSA) and the Girls Scout of the United States of America (GSUSA). Both groups offer badges in outdoor, craft, and industrial skills. But what badges teach a Scout about parenting and family life?

In the GSUSA, young women have been able to earn badges in Child Care, Cooking, and Home Health since the organization began in 1912. GSUSA has continued to develop badges in Family Living Skills, Family Financial Management, Healthy Relationships, Consumer Power, Sewing, and more.

The BSA, on the other hand, only began offering a Family Life merit badge in 1991. Currently, the number of Boy Scouts earning a Family Life merit badge is less than half the number of ones earning Woodworking, Archery, Fingerprinting, and any of the other merit badges, yet the Scouts with Family Life badges are far better off than the average young man.

Look around your network of friends and acquaintances. How many of them hire teenage boys to babysit their children if the boy isn't already a member of the family? How many use girl sitters instead? Very few boys get hands-on training in child-rearing—especially infant care. For example, when you were a boy, did you learn to change diapers? If you did, that's unusual. It's even more unusual if your father was the one who taught you to do it.

 Pregnant Pause

Don't let your lack of experience with infant care deter you. You can and will learn good ways to do this work and connect with your child.

Now think about what you learned from your father or stepfather about parenting. How much did he ever talk to you about how to be a father, or about how his life was enriched by having you as his son or stepson? This lack of words—father silence, if you will—is important for any new dad to acknowledge. Because you tend to start out with less training and information in fathering than your partner has in mothering, you have to recognize your need to reach out actively for knowledge.

That makes it essential to break this generational cycle of father silence. If you start talking about fathering—asking questions and sharing your experience—your own parenting will be better and easier. Other dads will benefit, too. The men you talk with will be ahead of the game. More importantly, your open discussion of fathering will give your own children words of wisdom they'll need when they take their turn as fathers and mothers.

Fathers could complain they were shortchanged as boys. Instead, I suggest recognizing there are things you need to learn now, and get on with finding ways to learn them. Then, if and when you have sons or grandsons of your own, you can make sure they get experience caring for infants and children.

Fathering Expectations

Fatherhood generates less conversation and attention in our society than motherhood does.

Nevertheless, you probably grew up knowing something about what people expect from fathers. For example, fathers are reliable, strong, and steady; they figure out problems and then fix them. They prepare themselves physically and psychologically to defend and direct their partners and children, especially in the world outside of home. And they do all of those things right.

If you think of these expectations as goals for you as a father, all are admirable. You can achieve them, but don't expect to achieve them perfectly and all the time. Flawless fathering isn't possible.

You can save yourself a lot of trouble and angst if you *don't* expect to be a perfect parent. Why not expect perfection?

- Because you won't be perfect (and neither is anyone else).

- Because you can be an excellent dad, even if you screw up sometimes.

- Because your child actually benefits from your mistakes and imperfections.

I worry about adults who expend enormous energy trying to parent perfectly. They seem to believe that any parental mistake will irreparably damage and scar their children.

However, that's not how mistakes work. In real life, we all screw up—because we're all imperfect. As protective parents, we sometimes forget that every mistake gives us a golden opportunity to learn something. Usually, the bigger the gaffe, the bigger the lesson to learn.

 Say, Dad

Mistakes are always forgivable, if one has the courage to admit them.

—Bruce Lee, martial artist and actor

Let's be clear: mistakes are no fun. They hurt. Your children may be hurt by their mistakes, and yours. However, hurt doesn't always equal harm. In fact, I'm willing to bet you learned some of life's most important lessons in the aftermath of a major flub.

You'll see an example of my favorite principle in action during the first year of your child's life. As your baby grows, he'll develop the urge to crawl. He'll want to get a toy (or extension cord) that's just out of his reach. But no matter how much he wants to crawl, he won't know how to do it at first. He'll learn to hold his back legs up and push his shoulders and head well off the ground. Meanwhile, his belly will remain anchored on the floor, and he won't be able to get going. He'll grunt, flap, rock his head, kick, and sometimes scream in frustration. He won't be happy. But after a few days or weeks, he'll somehow figure out how to crawl.

Will his frustration hurt him? No. While it may make him angry, it will also motivate him to motor himself across the floor.

Later on, after watching you stroll around the house, he'll begin to see that walking is faster and better than crawling. So he'll learn to stand up while holding onto your hands or a piece of furniture. In the process, he'll fall down—fairly often. He'll struggle as he learns how to get himself back upright again. He'll bang his head on the coffee table, get a bruise, and cry inconsolably. And once he figures out how to walk (and later, run), he will repeatedly lose him balance and fall down. Sometimes, as soon as he stands up, he'll topple over again.

Now, you could look at all this falling and head-bonking as a failure or mistake. They are! However, they are also opportunities to learn the skill—a universal example of trial and error.

Do we as fathers want our children to fall and hurt themselves? Of course not; it hurts us to see them hurt. But we understand these tenets:

- The baby will never learn to walk unless he falls down.
- Making the "mistake" of falling down hurts.
- The falling is still worth the effort.

Keep the thought of your baby learning to walk in mind during your years of fathering. Instead of instantly beating yourself up (or berating your child) over a blunder, recognize the other facets of making a mistake.

You and your child also need to learn that the consequences of mistakes are important lessons in responsibility. Remember to look for the other lessons and opportunities that human imperfections and errors provide, such as compassion, learning new skills, planning ahead, and so on.

The wonderful author and child psychologist Dr. David Walsh argues that so-called "helicopter parenting" harms kids. Hovering parents think that their job is to remove all the bumps in the road of their child's life (an impossibility). Dave says the more important job for you as a father is to equip your child with good shock absorbers so he learns to handle life's inevitable bumps and to bounce back from them.

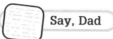 **Say, Dad**

Experience is merely the name men gave to their mistakes.

—Oscar Wilde, author

Dave's advice can be hard to follow. You don't want your children to be hurt by you or anyone else, and there will be times when you want to hover or rush in to rescue him from trouble—because you feel pain, too. However, "helicopter" parenting is not a good strategy. All of your child's fall-down-and-bonk "mistakes" eventually teach him to learn on his own.

Support and comfort him through the bumps, and then share in his pride. Remember that pride is an instinct that can also motivate and bolster *you* now and for years to come. Take pride in what you bring—and will bring—to your fatherhood.

The Veteran Dad

Remember those millennia worth of fathers who came before you? Quite a few of them are still around, so don't let them go to waste.

Let's suppose my four nearest neighbors and I added up the ages of all our respective children. For example, I have 34-year-old twins, so my number is 34 plus 34, or 68. Including the ages of the children from the other fathers, the collective grand total is over 250. So when we five men gather, there are more than two and a half centuries of fathering experience in the room. Plus, it's tough to come up with a situation one of us hasn't encountered. One dad has been married twice, one has a son with autism, one has twins, one had a child killed in a traffic accident, and two have grandchildren.

Despite this, few men actually talk to each other or to "veteran dads" about being a father. We're more comfortable discussing intricacies of our fantasy football league than the pros and cons of teaching an infant to swim.

 Attention, Please

You don't have to repeat strong-and-silent patterns in being your own man—or hang onto the discredited notion that "parenting is for women." You can ask questions and learn to develop your own style of parenting.

Pregnancy is a perfect time to use your courage and ask an experienced father for suggestions, advice, or wisdom. Or just ask him to tell stories about when he and his partner were pregnant. The odds that he'll be flattered (and happy to chat) are much better than the odds of winning at fantasy football.

And don't forget those veteran moms. Girls grow up hearing as much about parenting as we heard about sports. So when they grow up and become parents, they can also be valuable coaches for us rookies.

Your Dad and You

Your parents and stepparents may seem like a rich source of good ways to parent—or they may seem more like an endless example of how *not* to raise kids.

It's most likely, however, your parents did some things really well and some things rather poorly—with everything else falling somewhere in the middle. My kids would probably say that "in-between" is a good description of my own parenting.

When working with expectant dads, I encourage them to use these next few months to consider the kind of father they want to be. I'll talk about this more in Chapter 13, but a useful place to start is with a dispassionate appraisal of how the adults in your childhood parented you. I encourage those dads (and you) to do this simple activity:

- On a piece of paper, write down five good things your father, stepfather, or grandfather did that you want to be sure to do for your child.

- On a separate piece of paper, write down five things your father, stepfather, or grandfather did that you want to be sure to avoid doing to your child.

- Look over these lists both later in your partner's pregnancy and on your child's first birthday.

On the day your baby arrives, you'll learn how much improvising parenting involves. For example, rocking the baby to sleep with hip-hop music playing might work well for a week but then totally fail after that. Trial and error could lead you to a Johnny Mathis tune, and so you'll ride that wave until it peters out. The same pattern holds true as your child grows up; sometimes a strategy that works at one age may be a complete bust at another age.

Nevertheless, you might complain that your parents didn't recognize that you were too old (or too young) for strategy X and so they should have used strategy Y instead. Therefore, they didn't understand or respect you.

The truth is that, with a few rare exceptions, your parents were trying to do the right things. Like parents before and after their time, they had to improvise.

Getting this perspective can take a real load off as you realize the following:

- You parents didn't get an operating manual for you—and you're not getting one for your kid either.

- Working within their own limitations, most parents and stepparents do the best they can. (Sadly, a few parents don't do the best they can; they don't care or are cruel.)

- You are not your parents. You can take what you need from them and leave the rest.

It'll help you and your partner to remember that parenting is more art than science, no matter who's doing it. Nobody is or can be perfect (not you, your partner, your parents, your stepparents, your in-laws, or your child). Every one of your parents taught you at least one important lesson, even if it was the painful lesson of what not to do as a parent yourself. Be grateful and move forward.

 Attention, Please

You can probably identify relatives, friends, and acquaintances who grew up without one or the other of their parents due to death, incarceration, or other factors. As adults, some of those folks are doing fine and others not so well. No matter your parenting situation, you can make a huge contribution.

From my perspective, there's surprising value in reflecting on your parents' parenting. If you're like most men, you may give your dad more credit for doing well than you thought you might. Remember that when considering how much your dad and your other parents have to offer you along your fathering journey.

Finding Help Along the Way

If you're reading this book, you clearly want to be an involved and engaged father. That's very good news for you, your partner, and your offspring. So how do you get the information and guidance you wish you could find in a baby owner's manual that's good for all makes and models?

In addition to this book, here are other excellent sources of guidance:

Your gut. Nature has given parents the means to conceive, give birth to, and rear children for millennia. There's plenty of good animal instinct in your history and your genes, so don't be afraid to trust your gut. After all, there'd be no new child without your seminal participation, so you're connected tightly to your infant.

Your partner. You're in this together, so share the experience and communicate, communicate, communicate. Remember that human tools of communication include twice as many ears as mouths (in other words, listen more than you talk). Throughout this book, you'll see how much I emphasize the importance of communication.

Your family. They can be a great source of what to do in successful parenting … or what not to do (usually, both). As I said before, take what you need from your family history and leave the rest.

Other dads and moms. Yes, other parents are willing—even eager—to share their wisdom. Who doesn't like to be an expert? So talk (and listen) to veteran parents, especially the dads.

Fatherhood is a lot to handle, so take advantage of every resource you can reach!

The Least You Need to Know

- Be actively involved in raising your baby; it's good for the child and for you.
- Active fathering helps you, your partner, and your child.
- You can be a good father no matter how you were raised.
- Mistakes help your child grow, while hovering can inhibit child development.
- Veteran dads (and moms) are great resources for you.

CHAPTER 2

How to Get a Girl Pregnant

In This Chapter

- What health class left out
- How a sperm meets an egg
- Alternative ways to conceive
- Common conception myths

There's an old joke that goes like this: Why does it take 50 million sperm to fertilize one egg? Because they won't ask for directions either.

Strip away all the details, and getting pregnant boils down to two people having intercourse (an activity where stripping down makes things easier).

Or you may have to use other fertility options, such as in vitro fertilization (IVF), surrogate mothering, or other hormone therapies. Nevertheless, it's still wise to understand how pregnancy starts and progresses, as well as the layout of the plumbing that gets the baby rolling. I talk about that in this chapter, along with the common myths related to conception.

What High School Didn't Teach

Many schools still avoid (or water down) "sex education" because it's considered too controversial. Unfortunately, that leaves many kids without the most basic information about human reproduction.

To feel confident while you're expecting, and to be of the most use to your partner, it's important to know the basics of pregnancy.

 Say, Dad

Somewhere on this globe, every 10 seconds, there is a woman giving birth to a child. She must be found and stopped!

—Sam Levenson, comedian

In the flood of resources for expectant parents, you'll find many multi-syllabic words describing the various aspects of pregnancy. However, this amazing natural process starts simply enough.

Your Plumbing

Your reproductive organs start developing while you're still in the womb. At first, they look exactly like a female's organs. Soon, however, the two sexes' organs start to develop uniquely. For example, males don't begin making their reproductive cells (sperm) until they reach puberty, and they continue producing them into old age. A female is born with all the reproductive cells (eggs) she'll ever have; however, she doesn't start releasing them until puberty. If there are no health problems, she releases them every month until she reaches menopause.

The purpose of the male reproductive organs? To produce reproductive cells called *sperm*. They look like tadpoles, if you're peering through a super-strong microscope (or watching one of those grainy health-class films).

The reproductive process all starts in your testes (or testicles), those two small balls in your scrotum (the sac that hangs below your penis). One part of the teste produces androgen, the male hormone compound that includes testosterone. Androgen stimulates the other part of the teste to start forming sperm. You start making sperm in puberty and never stop. (I'll bypass speculation about any symbolism you attach to that fact and just say it's true.)

Sperm spend a lot of time in the pipelines and take a very roundabout trip through your body before jumping out. The testes have 750 feet of wound-tight tubes called the *epididymis* (there's one above each teste), which the sperm traverse before traveling into another coiled tube. Sperm "grow up" and get their tails in the epididymis and then hang around in storage until ejaculation.

When you get sexually stimulated, tiny muscles start pushing your sperm out the epididymis and through another tube called the *vas deferens*. This pipeline takes a more direct path while traveling north to make a big circle next to your bladder. The vas deferens deposits the sperm into the seminal vesicles, where they pick up seminal fluid to feed the sperm and give them something in which to "spread their tails" and start swimming. Exhausted yet?

Your sperm then move down into the prostate gland, which secretes a milky fluid into your urethra (hang in there, I'll tell you what a urethra is in a second), so your sperm can really cut loose for a swim. Just below the prostate are the two Cowper's glands, which send a fluid into the urethra to facilitate the sperms' swimming journey. The urethra (drum roll, please) is the tube in your penis through which semen (the combination of all this fluid and sperm) passes.

 Attention, Please

Your urine also passes out of the urethra, but never at the same time as your semen. A series of muscles act as gates to let only one or the other through.

Surrounding the urethra are tissues called *corpus cavernosa* and *corpus spongiosum*, poetic Latin terms that suggest caverns and sponges. Basically, these caverns and sponges fill with blood when you get aroused during sexual activity, expanding your penis into an erection. The erection later collapses when blood leaves your corpus cavernosa and corpus spongiosum and goes back where it came from.

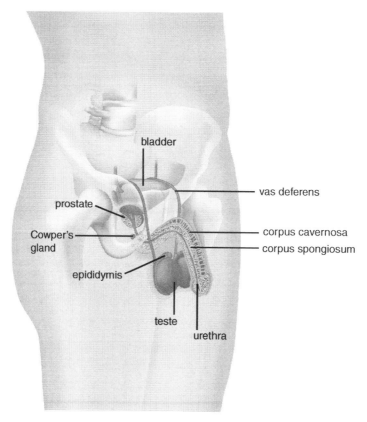

When all systems are working normally, a muscle below your prostate gland will "open the gate" and let the semen into your urethra. The combination of the blood coursing through your penis and other muscle action causes the semen to rush (or ejaculate) through the urethra and out the opening at the end of your penis.

If you look at the diagram, the whole process doesn't seem very efficient. It starts in your testes, which are millimeters from the tip of your penis. But the sperm first have to travel in a long route (almost a figure eight) before they gather up all their tools, leave "home," and leap out of your penis.

If the tip of your penis is inside (or even close to, as health teachers and preachers like to remind you) the vagina of a fertile female at ejaculation, pregnancy is possible. As far as the biology of pregnancy goes, the rest is up to your sperm and the plumbing of your partner.

Her Plumbing

A female's reproductive system invests far more time (36 to 39 weeks) on a pregnancy than the male's system does (36 to 39 seconds?). However, the female's plumbing is more straightforward—it has a lot fewer tubes, at any rate.

The visible part of your partner's reproductive organs is the vulva, which includes the labia majora and labia minora. These cover and protect the vagina, urethra, and clitoris. In a woman, the urethra only carries urine (nothing else), and the only purpose of the clitoris (a *very* important one) is to give sexual pleasure to the woman.

For this discussion, the vagina is top priority. The vagina is a moist, flexible tunnel that starts at the vulva and ends 4 or more inches inside the body at the cervix. It holds the penis during intercourse and is where the sperm go when they leave you.

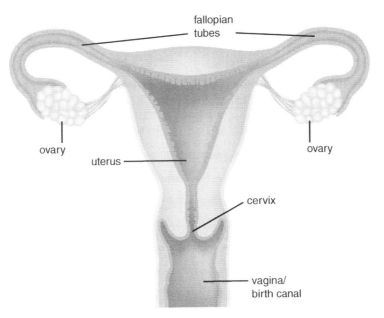

On the other side of the cervix is the uterus, which is about 3 inches long when a woman isn't pregnant. The versatile uterus is very flexible and gets much bigger when she is pregnant.

For a sperm to trigger the start of a pregnancy, it has to pass through the cervix and travel all the way up the uterus to the tiny opening of a fallopian tube (see, they do have *some* tubes). A woman has two fallopian tubes on the "north" end of the uterus—one coming in from the west and the other from the east. Each fallopian tube forms a 3½-inch circular path between the uterus and an ovary.

There's one ovary on each side of a female—right under the point halfway between the top of her leg and her belly button. The two ovaries house the million or so unfertilized eggs a woman has from birth. As I mentioned earlier, she doesn't produce any more eggs during her lifetime. However, in most cases, her body will bring one egg to maturation each month between puberty and menopause while immature eggs hang out in follicles inside the ovaries.

The ovaries also generate female hormones, such as estrogen, that facilitate the menstruation and pregnancy cycles. These hormones stimulate the follicles, and each month an egg matures, cuts loose, and is pushed out of the ovary. At this point, a fallopian tube can snag the egg and muscle it along to the uterus.

If a sperm and an egg get together, they "do it" in a fallopian tube. That spot sounds so romantic; you have to wonder why neither Shakespeare nor Taylor Swift ever wrote a ballad called "Under the Fallopian Moon."

 Say, Dad

Whoever called it necking was a poor judge of anatomy.

—Groucho Marx, comedian

If Sperm Played Baseball

When you ejaculate, you send out tens of millions of sperm. But before you start thinking too highly of yourself (or your sperm), remember this: sperm are a lot like lemmings. In order to reach the female's egg, one of those 50 to 250 million sperm must travel only about 6 inches (15 centimeters). However, 15 centimeters is nearly 4,000 times the length of a sperm cell. If a single sperm were the size of a human, it would have to swim a complicated 40-mile route to reach the woman's fertile egg—while battling a field of competitors larger than the population of Japan.

Most of the time, none of your sperm are up to the job. Their cumulative batting average wouldn't even qualify for a Little League team. But a miraculous chain reaction begins that one time when a successful sperm reaches the egg, passes through the egg's wall, and fertilizes it. This is the moment of conception.

The combined sperm and egg are called the *zygote*. All of the genetic information and material your baby will ever have is right there in the zygote from the beginning, even though it's only about one tenth of a millimeter long.

 Baby Steps

You can get a positive pregnancy test as early as 7 to 10 days after conception, even before your partner notices she has missed a period.

Within a couple weeks, the fallopian tube pushes the zygote down into the uterus. (Pushing is a recurring theme in pregnancy.) If a number of things progress exactly as planned, the zygote then attaches itself to the endometrium, a lush lining of tissue and blood along the wall of the uterus. If no zygote attaches to the endometrium, it deteriorates and is flushed out of the uterus in the monthly process known as menstruation, or "having a period."

Once the zygote latches onto the uterine wall, pregnancy begins, and the zygote becomes an embryo. During pregnancy, an embryo remains an embryo until all of its major organs have developed. After that point—usually about four months into the pregnancy— your baby is called a *fetus*.

Your Health and Hers

Expecting a baby is physically and mentally stressful for you and your partner. You both face some big unknowns, as well as the excitement of creating a new life, which can generate stress. The antidote for stress is active and conscious care of your body and your spirit.

Communicate, Communicate, Communicate

Unfortunately, many men have learned unhealthy "responses" to stress. We think showing any weakness or asking for help is impotent, wrong, and wimpy. Jackson Katz, author and consultant for the U.S. Air Force and Defense Department, calls this mistaken strategy an example of putting on our "Tough Guise." Paradoxically, successful dads find that things go far better when they ask for help and guidance with their fathering and that being "vulnerable" is one of the greatest challenges and joys of fathering.

It's a common mistake to see vulnerability as evidence of weakness. In fact, it's evidence of courage, strength, and belief in one's self. Vulnerability opens doors through which you can bond with your partner and your children, giving you the *strongest* human connections you may ever have.

The first step in keeping your spirits up under stress is to communicate with your partner, family, friends, and health-care professionals. Let them know what you need, what you're thinking, and what you're feeling. (Yes, even what you're feeling!) Open communication unlocks the psychological pressure valves and makes it easier to tune into the good, exciting, and energizing things happening in your pregnancy. And those regular doses of exhilaration will give you energy and adrenaline to carry you through the stresses of expecting—and even labor and delivery!

When it comes to your partner's emotional health, remember the value of an occasional and strategic white lie. No, you shouldn't pretend that green is blue (I never pretend; I'm colorblind and can't tell the difference!), nor should you stifle important thoughts and feelings. But there are occasions when you help your cause—and ease your partner's stress—by delivering a "Yes, dear" or a "No, you look fabulous," even if that's not your genuine sentiment at the moment. The keyword is *strategic*. This is one time when less is more in a loving relationship. You don't want to get yourself into jams requiring a white lie so often that you develop bad habits. However, an occasional, considerate "fib" can make both of you feel better.

Finally, to help you both have a less-stressful experience, throw resentment out of your expectant dad's toolbox and don't let it back in. For example, you may be tempted to feel resentful when she gets all the attention and you seem to be ignored. But choosing resentment as a tool to respond is bound to jam your gears.

Pregnant Pause

Resentment never delivers on its "I'll show you!" promise. Author Elizabeth Gilbert compares resentment to smoking: "Even one puff is bad for you."

Resentment eats away at the resentor long before it has much impact (if any) on the resentee. When you resent something that's happening, the first person you undermine is yourself. Plus, resentment never changes the problem. Change comes from action and constructive attitudes.

Instead of resentment, try showing kindness to your partner, even if you're struggling with her at the moment. You can also make a short gratitude list of five things you appreciate in life every night before you go to sleep. The most effective antidote for resentment is gratitude; do it for a few nights, and you'll feel the difference.

Bottom line? If an expectant dad is resentful, then he can expect nothing but trouble. So do yourself a favor, and don't go there.

Your Body Counts, Too

You know a pregnant woman has to take care of her body in order to have a good pregnancy and increase the odds of a healthy baby—that means getting moderate exercise; eating wisely; and abstaining from alcohol, drugs, tobacco, and other harmful substances. But pregnancy is also an excellent time for you to pay attention to your own health. Improving your physical and mental condition will improve your energy, focus, and stamina, which are important resources for the rest of this pregnancy and beyond.

Physical activity brings concrete benefits to your body and spirit. The new demands of expecting (and, eventually, parenting) may translate into less time on the bike or basketball court, but don't give up on it altogether. Being active is more effective (and much better for your health) than alternatives like tobacco and alcohol. In addition to helping to relieve stress, exercise keeps you in better touch with your body.

When it comes to nutrition, think of this common computer programmer saying: garbage in, garbage out. Eating healthy improves your health and longevity. In addition to the personal benefits, your child will enjoy you more if you're in good health and live longer! It can also save your relationship with your partner, especially if she has to follow special nutritional guidelines during pregnancy. You're going to look (and be) rather rude eating a banana split while she works through a spinach salad. Would you resent that behavior if the kitchen tables were turned? Remember that neither one of you is a saint, so support—and join in with—the meals she needs to keep the pregnancy on track.

Like exercise, good nutrition also strengthens your connection to your body. Why the focus on staying attuned to your body? During pregnancy, your partner invests a lot of energy and focus on tracking what's happening in (and to) her body. If you invest a bit in your own body, you increase your ability to empathize with and support her. That investment also sharpens your thinking, making you a better observer and problem solver.

When Nature Won't Cooperate

So far, I've described the process of a relatively ordinary pregnancy, when nature's systems work as they are expected to. However, there are times when—through no fault of your own—the "usual" way of getting pregnant doesn't work so smoothly. Fortunately, there are other ways to bring a child into your life and home, including artificial insemination, surrogacy, and adoption.

Missed Conceptions: Infertility

In the United States, around 10 percent of couples encounter fertility problems of one sort or another. Disruption of the woman's ability to ovulate (known as *anovulation*) is a common issue in infertility. The pituitary gland or hypothalamus may malfunction, throwing off the hormone balance needed to produce fertile eggs. The ovary may be scarred or the follicles may not break open to release the egg.

Anovulation isn't the only problem. Excessive growth of the uterine lining (endometriosis), polyps, cysts, tumors, or congenital problems can inhibit or prevent the uterus from hosting a successful pregnancy.

The fallopian tubes may be blocked, scarred, or infected. The mucus on the cervix may not have the right consistency or abundance to help move sperm along.

Male infertility stems from hormonal imbalance, disease, congenital defects, and lifestyle choices. As with women, disruptions in the hypothalamus, thyroid, or pituitary glands can foul up the hormone balance your sperm need to work effectively. Variocoele (basically, varicose veins in the scrotum), erectile dysfunction, premature ejaculation, damaged sperm ducts, infection, and other fairly rare conditions can also inhibit male fertility.

To discover the underlying problem, doctors will analyze your semen and test your partner's ovary, cervix, and other organs for issues with their structure and functioning.

However, some fertility problems go beyond the physical. Your behavior can have a major impact on whether you and your partner conceive. If you want to have a baby, medical researchers say you should avoid the following:

- Alcohol abuse

- Smoking

- Anabolic steroids

- "Recreational" drugs, including marijuana

- Exposure to environmental hazards, such as toxic chemicals and radioactivity

- Overexercising

- Lack of sleep

- Excess stress

Many responses to infertility focus solely on the female, often because women are more likely to seek medical care and guidance than men. If you two have trouble getting pregnant, don't be average—be part of the solution from day one.

Infertility Options

Because hormone imbalance is a common culprit for the man and woman, your doctors may prescribe synthetic hormone drugs (a.k.a. hormone replacement therapy) for one or both of you. It can take a few months for hormone levels to reach the necessary levels in the body, so be patient. In fact, patience is an essential habit when dealing with infertility.

Doctors can use a wide variety of drugs (with different "brand" and generic names), so be sure you discuss these options thoroughly with each other and your medical professionals. Hormone replacement therapy can also produce side effects, so be sure you have good knowledge of these potential effects before deciding on a course of treatment.

Your doctors may also recommend surgery to correct some issues related to structural problems in reproductive organs. Some procedures aim to unblock obstructions, while other procedures work to bypass the obstructions and surgically insert semen into the uterus. In men, surgery can often correct problems with varicocele and blocked ducts.

Sex as a Chore

More treatments for infertility are available than ever before—and nearly all of them are stressful. Perhaps the biggest stressor is the way you may now have to engage in sex. Many couples getting infertility treatment say the prescribed regimen for intercourse and other sexual acts is a major adjustment. After all, you're both probably used to having sex spontaneously because you're in the mood, not because you're on a timetable.

As part of fertility treatments, you may have to ejaculate in a doctor's office or laboratory. Your partner may need pelvic exams, shots, and other intrusive (and painful) procedures. Hormone therapy can affect your mood and libido. Not to mention how you and your partner have to refrain from or engage in intercourse on a physician-designed schedule. In addition, infertility treatments are time-consuming and expensive.

Worst of all, you may feel like less of a man—and your partner less of a woman—because you're having trouble getting pregnant. All this can take a toll on your sex life—and your whole relationship.

 Attention, Please

Feeling "infertile" can challenge some core parts of your identity, which makes it even more essential that you and your partner trust each other, remain honest, and pull together.

Here are some steps—not necessarily easy—to help you if sex begins to feel like a chore or an assault on your self-worth:

- **Be gentle with yourself.** Pamper your mood and your body.

- **Be gentle with your partner.** Remember (and remind her of) how sexy and attractive she is, inside and out.

- **Go beyond intercourse.** Cuddling, snuggling, or giving each other space can be great comforts—and build intimacy between you.

- **Act the part.** Feelings often follow behavior, so don't be afraid to "act" sexy even when you don't necessarily feel sexy. As the old saying goes, fake it until you make it.

- **Use some ritual.** Develop some routines to set a mood using things like candles, erotica, good music, and so on. Go on dates, pretending you're just beginning your relationship. Experiment to find things that work for you both.

- **Communicate.** This experience is an opportunity to know yourself and your partner better. That also makes it an opportunity to draw closer together. Keep listening and keep sharing, and you'll make it through this together.

Will We Have to Call Him Beaker?

If intercourse can't produce a pregnancy, you might consider assisted reproductive technology (ART), the term physicians use to cover a number of methodologies. One widely recognized procedure is artificial insemination, known as intrauterine insemination (IUI) in the medical field. Your partner is likely to be given drugs to stimulate ovulation before the procedure. During the IUI procedure, you ejaculate semen into a container. The doctor then injects this semen into the uterus or fallopian tube of your partner.

Another well-known method is in vitro fertilization (IVF), which (unlike IUI) requires removing the woman's eggs from her ovaries and mixing them with the man's sperm in a laboratory. Afterward, the doctor inserts the embryos back into her body, with the goal of having embryonic development proceed naturally from there. IVF also involves hormone replacement drugs to stimulate your partner's ovaries.

Ideally, the sperm used in IVF are your own. If there are problems with your sperm, however, you may decide to use a donor. Likewise, if your partner can't produce fertile eggs, you can decide to use an egg donor. Whatever the case, the sperm or eggs can be used right away or frozen for later use. IVF and IUI can (and often do) take more than one cycle to take hold. It will be an up-and-down journey, so be patient.

Mike Moore, creator of the Husband's IVF Journey blog (hubbyivf-journey.blogspot.com), and his wife gave birth to their daughter in 2011 after using IVF. Mike describes IVF as "one of the most fantastic, nerve-wracking, emotion-stirring, relationship-strengthening things we have *ever* been through." For example, as their first egg-retrieval day approached, Mike was calm and cool on the outside. But inside, he says, "I felt like I was a week out from Christmas."

Mike suggests doing the following if you decide to go the IVF route:

- Never be shy about asking questions.

- Be respectful, but never let medical staffers bully you.

- Build a relationship with the receptionist at the doctor's office—you never know when you'll need to cash in some IOUs.

- Check message boards and websites "occasionally" for validation, but don't rely solely on them for all of your information.

- Make sure you spend some time out of the house. The walls tend to close in as you wait on different phases of the process.

- Don't let another couple's less-than-positive experience impact yours. Pray, love, and smile when you can; it does wonders for the soul.

Surrogacy

If ART doesn't produce a pregnancy, some couples turn to a surrogate. That's a woman who's able and willing to accept an embryo into her uterus and carry the pregnancy through to the end. At delivery, the baby goes to the "intended" parents—you and your partner.

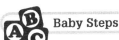 **Baby Steps**

Depending on the circumstances, you can use your partner's eggs, a donor's eggs, or the surrogate's own eggs.

Tabloids and websites are filled with stories of surrogacy arrangements gone wrong. However, reality suggests that such problems are the exception.

Research shows that surrogate mothers rarely struggle to relinquish rights to a surrogate child; in fact, a large majority feel empowered by the experience. The surrogate's own children (in other words, the ones she raises) don't usually suffer any negative impact either.

Furthermore, researchers from City University London (UK) found that, when compared to "natural conception" parents, intended fathers had lower levels of parental stress and intended moms showed more positive parent-child relationships when the baby was born via surrogate.

Some surrogate mothers carry the pregnancy for money and others volunteer. Either way, you and your partner need to make a legally binding agreement with the surrogate mother and rely on reputable agencies to help you through this expensive process.

As with other aspects of pregnancy, surrogacy will stir up its share of questions, fears, and emotions, so discuss it with each other and your family and friends honestly and lovingly.

Adoption

According to the National Adoption Information Clearinghouse (adoption.org), adoption is "the permanent legal transfer of parenting rights and responsibilities from one family to another." More than 125,000 children are adopted in the United States each year, and the number of foreign-born children adopted by U.S. families continues to grow.

Adoption brings a child born to other parents into your life and family. The reasons someone gives up a child for adoption are complex. But for most birth parents, the central reason is wanting the child to have a better life than they feel they can provide.

Adopted children come from orphanages, foster care, or through arrangements with a pregnant birth mother or her family. Infants can be more difficult to adopt than older babies or children, because there's more demand for infant adoptions.

If you live in the United States, you have multiple options for adopting a child born in the country, also known as a *domestic adoption:*

* Licensed public agencies, which usually handle adoption of children in foster care.

* Licensed private agencies, which work directly with the birth parents to arrange an adoption.

* Independent adoption, where the adoptive parents identify a birth mother and then work with an attorney to arrange the adoption. These arrangements must be approved by a court.

- Facilitators and unlicensed agencies who work to match adopting parents with birth mothers for a fee. However, they may have little or no oversight or expertise. In fact, some states prohibit adoptions by paid facilitators.

Most jurisdictions require court approval of the adoption, no matter who facilitates it. In addition, U.S. law makes it more complex to adopt a child who's enrolled (or could be enrolled) in an Indian tribe.

Foreign or "intercountry" adoption varies depending on the agency you choose, the child's country of origin, and whether or not the country is one of the 75 signers of the Hague Convention on Protection of Children and Co-operation in Respect of Intercountry Adoption. You can find more information on intercountry adoption at childwelfare.gov/pubs/factsheets/hague.cfm.

 Say, Dad

I am not ashamed to say that no man I ever met was my father's equal, and I never loved any other man as much.

—Hedy Lamarr, actress and inventor

Learn as much as possible about the child's background and health—for example, whether she has Fetal Alcohol Syndrome. Health conditions may not be apparent if the child is an infant, so extensive knowledge about birth parents and their circumstances helps.

For all its benefits, adoption can still be strange or startling to some people. When you tell family and friends you're adopting, you may encounter uninformed questions (such as "How will your 'real' children feel?") or even blatantly bigoted attitudes (especially if you're adopting from overseas). You need a plan to discuss the adoption that does the following:

- Addresses misconceptions and prejudiced comments directly

- Takes advantage of every opportunity to teach others about adoption

- Shows patience with people who may not know as much as you do about adoption

- Allows you to decide how much information you're willing to share

- Is sensitive to the mixed feelings some relatives may have

It's important to develop, use, and modify this plan now because you'll need it when you meet new people throughout your baby's childhood. Plus, in later years, your child will probably be listening in when you respond to these inevitable questions.

 Pregnant Pause

Some relatives may not immediately jump for joy at the news that you're adopting. For example, your parents may struggle with feelings (and even grief) that their genetic heritage won't be passed on or that this won't be a "real" grandchild. Anticipate these reactions and prepare to reassure your loved one. And jump for joy if they're as excited as you are!

In the end, you don't need to worry too much, because parents and other relatives usually get over these feelings pretty quickly. So don't take their feelings personally, and be patient. Your sensitivity will help hasten the time when Grandma is excited about the idea of your child, regardless of what womb she came from.

Above all, make sure you're clear and comfortable with your feelings about welcoming your child into your family. Your clarity makes it easier for relatives and friends and gives you a better foundation for confronting any challenges that arise now or later.

The Birds, the Bees, and the Bull

Getting pregnant and giving birth has been around for a very long time. Even with all the scientific advancement, some moldy old myths still linger on. I close with some here, with the hope they offer you a bit of comic relief.

Sunshine, Gravity, and Lubrication

Some research suggests that a man's sperm levels are slightly higher during the daytime, leading to the myth that making love during the daytime improves your chances of getting pregnant. However, that slight increase in sperm levels doesn't really make a difference—after all, we're talking hundreds of millions of sperm.

Another myth is that drinking cough syrup thins mucus on the woman's cervix the same way it does in your bronchia, leading to easier conception. Nope, it doesn't help.

Same thing with the belief that vaginal lubricants improve fertility by supplementing cervical mucus. In fact, most lubricants tend to upset the chemical environment in the vagina and can kill sperm. If you'd like to know more about lubricants and their effect on fertility, check with your doctor.

Gravity isn't a lot of help either, so don't buy in to the myths about you or your partner needing to contort your bodies for conception. For example, if your partner lies on her back with her legs in the air after intercourse, it doesn't help the sperms' journey—there are too many twists, turns, and obstacles in the way. (Our reproductive systems have learned to work around gravity anyway.)

Ice in Your Boxers

Will your sperm count increase if you put ice in your pants? Cooler temperatures can slightly increase sperm production—but only after about two months. So an ice pack won't help.

Green tea (iced or hot) is sometimes touted as fabulous for fertility. It does have some health benefits and has less fertility-unfriendly caffeine than other teas, but there's no clinical connection between green tea and your chances of a healthy pregnancy.

Other "cooling" solutions—such as wearing boxers instead of briefs (increases airflow!) or avoiding saunas, hot tubs, or hot showers—also don't improve the chances of conceiving.

Bikes, Bananas, and Boys

Riding bikes and running produce genital heat, not to mention bouncing and bumping the testicles, but there's no evidence that exercise affects your sperm output. In fact, moderate exercise is good for both of you and doesn't affect conception.

Another myth is that men who eat nonorganic bananas will be sterile. Farm chemicals can impact the health (including fertility) of farm workers, but a few bananas shouldn't harm your sperm count.

Perhaps the most stubborn pregnancy myth is the one suggesting you can predetermine your baby's gender by conceiving early (a boy) or later (a girl) in your partner's fertile cycle. Not only is this false, but limiting the intercourse you have during fertile periods can cut down the odds of getting pregnant.

Orgasmic, Daily, or Underwater Sex?

A female orgasm sets off contractions in the uterus. Therefore, those contractions should push the sperm closer to the fallopian tubes, right? Well …. Orgasms may have some slight effect on sperm movement, but not enough to make it the determining factor in whether you and your partner conceive. But let's be clear: an orgasm is a good thing in and of itself—no other motivation is needed! So be a loving and communicative partner and help her achieve orgasm as often as she likes.

 Attention, Please

No sexual position has been shown to increase the prospect of getting pregnant. Nature has her ways, and shifting positions doesn't seem to help. Therefore, find the most comfortable positions for you both; if it feels good, you'll do it more.

Daily intercourse can be fun if you both like it, but quantity alone doesn't get your partner pregnant. That requires having sex during her fertile period. But hey, there's no reason to avoid making love the rest of the time!

Some people believe that having sex in a pool or hot tub increases the chances of fertility, because the water helps the sperm swim upstream. Others believe that water interferes with cervical mucus and therefore works as a contraceptive. And still others think that the heat of a hot tub will kill off enough sperm to affect conception. There's no clinical evidence to support any of those claims. If you like making love in the water, go for it, but it's not shown to positively or negatively affect the ability to conceive.

Other Popular Myths

Just for fun, let's debunk a few more myths:

- A woman can't get pregnant if she's never had sex before. (Oh, yes she can.)

- If the guy pulls out before ejaculating, the girl can't get pregnant. (Oops, there's also sperm in the preejaculation lubricant secreted by the penis.)

- She can't get pregnant if she sneezes after sex. (No sneeze has the power to eject semen, and our species propagates even when Momma has a cold.)

- If you take one of her birth control pills right before sex, she won't get pregnant. (Absolute wishful thinking.)

The Least You Need to Know

- Male and female reproductive organs are miraculous but not completely mysterious.
- If you have fertility problems, you can explore other ways to become parents, such as hormone treatments or surrogacy.
- Fertility treatments and adoption require patience, understanding, and extra communication effort.
- Separating the facts from the myths about pregnancy can keep you grounded and help ready you to be a dad.

Sex During Pregnancy

In This Chapter

- Separating pregnancy sex myth and fact
- Hormonal changes during pregnancy that affect your sex life
- Learning to love the bump
- Having sex after your baby's born

Your partner will change in appearance, attention, and mood during her pregnancy. You may wonder (and worry) about these changes—especially how they will impact your sex life.

Will your partner still be interested in you? Will you still be interested in her? Is it possible, practical, or safe to have sex while she's pregnant? And will either one of you want to? What about sex after pregnancy—how will it be different? In this chapter, I provide you the answers to all these questions and more.

Facts About Pregnancy Sex

Let's start by dispelling some lingering urban myths about sex during pregnancy.

Sex does *not* increase chances of a miscarriage. Nature accounts for the fact that most partners will still have sex after conception; it keeps the baby well protected. The combination of amniotic fluid holding the baby and the strong muscles surrounding the uterus provide a substantial safety cushion.

Intercourse will *not* hurt the baby or your partner. As I mentioned in the previous paragraph, your baby is very protected during the pregnancy. As for your partner, intercourse won't hurt if you work together (especially as she gets bigger) to use sexual positions that don't strain her body or cause her pain. I'll say more on that later in this chapter.

It will *not* bring on premature labor. Later in the pregnancy, the production of oxytocin (a hormone that stimulates contractions) may accelerate during foreplay with your partner's breasts. However, as you'll learn in childbirth class (and in Chapter 6), many women have small and safe contractions for a while before they go into full-fledged labor.

 Pregnant Pause

Don't have sex if your partner's water has broken—or, in medical lingo, once the membrane around the baby's amniotic sac has ruptured. In fact, if the sac breaks, you should be on the phone with the doctor or on the way to the hospital, preparing to welcome a new kind of whoopee!

Oral sex is fine during pregnancy. It won't trigger anything dangerous, and it's a fun alternative to intercourse as her body changes. One caveat: don't blow air directly into her vagina. That could cause a dangerous air bubble in the bloodstream.

Bump Sex and Hormones

As the pregnancy progresses and her belly grows, it's harder to reach familiar places in the old familiar ways. Intercourse will require several adjustments (and perhaps a few laughs) as you try to devise workable methods.

Throughout it all, her hormones will be on the march and her body working overtime to grow another person. Your hormones and attitudes are in flux, too, so it's smart to stay flexible and consider the many changes your partner is going through as you discuss and think about being sexually intimate.

Dancing with the Hormones

You've probably heard that pregnancy brings major hormonal changes to your partner's body (see more about hormones in general in Chapter 4). The most famous symptom of pregnancy due to hormones is euphemistically known as "morning sickness." Spoiler alert: your partner's nausea and vomiting will happen at all hours of the day and night. These are certified romantic turnoffs, but they usually pass by the end of the first trimester for most women.

 Say, Dad

You don't have to be the Dalai Lama to tell people that life's about change.

—John Cleese, comedian

If she's like most pregnant women, your partner will also have ups and downs in her energy level and her libido over the course of these nine months due to hormones. As I'll explain throughout the book, pregnancy creates huge changes in her body and can exhaust her. Since a person needs some energy to be interested in sex, her desire may go up and down, too … and not necessarily on the same schedule as your desire.

Another libido inhibitor can be the realization that she's becoming a mother. Psychologically, it can be hard to reconcile motherhood with her sense of her sexuality. Do motherhood and sex go together? I mean, can you imagine your mother (or mother-in-law) ever having sex? (Spoiler alert 2: … oh, never mind.) This emotional struggle may not be logical, but it is real, and changes in hormone levels can bring those emotions to the forefront.

Fortunately for most women, pregnancy also brings bursts of physical and emotional energy based on hormonal changes. When it comes to lovemaking, some of that energy comes from the liberating feeling flowing from the knowledge that sex can't get her pregnant. That knowledge can liberate you, too.

With those bursts of energy and freedom, she may think about sex more often than normal and want you to have sex with her more frequently. Again, however, these times are likely to come and go over the course of her pregnancy.

Your partner may also be among those women whose sex drive doesn't accelerate during pregnancy. This is not a sign of failure on her part or yours. It also doesn't mean your relationship is in trouble or that she doesn't love you anymore. It just means that pregnancy, hormones, and other changes are running how her psyche and body feel.

The uncertainty can be a problem, but it is certainly also an opportunity to openly, kindly, and mutually discuss your feelings and beliefs about sex and sexuality. Encourage and invite those conversations—you'll learn a lot about each other. That knowledge has great potential to bring you closer together.

Everyone has convictions, anxieties, hopes, and fears about sexuality—their own and their partner's. The changes of pregnancy tend to bring these to the surface, as you deal with the psychological adjustments you both go through as you approach parenthood. So don't avoid the topic; listen closely, take your partner seriously, and learn from what you hear.

Remember that sexuality is *one* aspect of your relationship with each other, not its entirety. She still needs you, so dive into other ways of connecting with each other. Meanwhile, don't lose hope; her hormones may yet send her into another gear where she can't wait to go to bed with you.

And before long, the baby will be here, and your partner's hormones will (eventually) become less volatile.

Daddy's Hormones

Among my favorite photos of my wife are ones from the 36 hours after our children were born. There was a vibrancy about her, as if some special light was actually shining through her skin. I felt awe about that sensation on the days it happened, and I still feel it when I see the photos more than 30 years later.

Could it be that nature creates a pregnant woman's luminescent skin and plump body in order to capture her mate's attention and stimulate his pride? After all, her pregnant body is a vibrant sign of you virility—a sign the whole world can see.

Her appearance is, of course, also a sign of her fertility, which can be very attractive to other men. Don't be surprised if guys flirt with her at a party, in the parking lot, or in the produce aisle. It seems natural for men to feel drawn to a voluptuous woman.

In fact, it *is* natural. Pheromones secreting from a pregnant woman may be an evolutionary adaptation that works to attract members of the opposite sex. However, these mysterious chemicals have more impact on you than any other people—because the amount of time you spend with her gives you more pheromone exposure.

 Attention, Please

Your partner's pregnancy may affect how your pets respond to her. Cats tend to avoid pregnant women, while dogs tend to get more protective of them. This may be a result of your partner's pheromones.

Pheromones also appear to increase the expectant father's level of prolactin (a "female" hormone that helps trigger lactation in your partner) and lower your testosterone levels slightly. This may be nature's way to bring you greater feelings of desire for your partner and a greater urge to protect her (and the baby). Think of it as another way that the legacy of fathers aligns your moods, attitudes, and perspective with becoming a dad.

So be proud of how hot she looks; it's working for you!

Physical Changes

You've been making your way through the world since the day you were born. Along the way, you've no doubt noticed that women's bodies look different when they're pregnant. However, you may not know how pregnancy affects a woman internally and changes her sexual experiences.

Luscious and Sensitive

In order to sustain and grow the fetus, a pregnant woman's blood flow increases substantially. This extra blood engorges (to use the medical term) many parts of her body, especially the parts related to childbirth and lactation.

Most pregnant women see their breasts grow in size as hormones prepare breast tissue to feed the newborn. (You'll see this, too!) Her vagina and clitoris also increase in sensitivity thanks to engorgement, as her body loosens and lubricates that area in order to ease the way for baby's birth.

For many women, this "juicier" appearance broadcasts her desirability, which is great for her ego and makes her sexual appetite increase. Research also suggests that women have an easier time achieving—and maintaining—orgasm during pregnancy. It's wonderful to give your partner such pleasure because it tends to increase your sexual pleasure while stimulating greater psychological and emotional intimacy between you. Plus, it's fun!

Be aware, however, that your partner's breasts, vagina, and clitoris may be sensitive to any kind of touch or sensation, particularly during the first trimester. Sometimes, even foreplay and sex that causes great pleasure can suddenly cross the line into pain. Be patient, and follow her lead and desires to learn what feels good for her.

Don't worry if you're sometimes out of breath trying to keep pace with her sexual appetite. Giving her pleasure helps her feel great, which is a bonus for your relationship, her health, and the baby. They key is directing your intimacy and sexual activity toward building love and joy in your relationship.

Attention, Please

Even though the clitoris is right next the vagina, it doesn't have a direct role in reproduction. Its only function is to stimulate orgasm and provide sexual pleasure for women. An outstanding purpose on its own, clitoral pleasure is an incentive for women to have sex, giving this special organ an indirect role in perpetuating the species.

More to Love

Women gain weight during pregnancy, thank goodness. They also need a higher percentage of body fat to be healthy than men do.

Before puberty, a girl's body has about 12 percent body fat. During puberty, nature's hardwiring increases the number of fat cells to about 17 percent of her body, making it possible for her to safely ovulate and menstruate. If the girl's growth is natural (and uninterrupted by dieting), her mature adult body will have about 22 percent body fat.

 Attention, Please

Through the hardwiring of their bodies, pregnant women can survive a food shortage long enough to give birth. In this way, nature assures propagation of the human species even during famine. Nature also assures that women gain fat first in the breasts, buttocks, hips, and thighs after puberty, which helps protect the female reproductive organs and ensure lactation.

Now that your partner's body is functioning for two, it needs space for the baby and fat cells to nourish baby and her. Fat cells in the breasts multiply as they prepare to feed the child once he's born.

In other words, fat is fabulous right now.

Unfortunately, it may not be fabulous for other people in a culture that tends to despise fat and fat people. As humorist Dave Barry says in his tongue-in-cheek rules for life, "You should never say anything to a woman that even remotely suggests that you think she's pregnant unless you can see an actual baby emerging from her at that moment." If neither of you have naturally large bodies, social prejudice about large bodies may come as a shock as your partner grows. Therefore, pregnancy can be a good time for both of you to think about the social taboo against fat.

Scientific research makes clear that it's possible to be healthy at a wide variety of body shapes and sizes, so don't fall into the trap of conflating weight and health. Remember, too, that she may have more of *you* to love. Some researchers find that the average expectant dad also gains weight after the first trimester. This could be due to meal servings getting larger to compensate for your partner and baby, joining her in daily "grazing," or even adding sympathy pounds. In other words, there's likely to be more for each of you to love.

Think of weight gain as good practice for the baby's arrival, when you and your partner can feel another big expansion of love. In addition, remind your partner—and yourself—that women's bodies act this way for a *very* good reason. Tell her how amazing her pregnant body is. And more important, feel free to *show* her how much you like it, too.

Variety Is the Spice of Life

During most pregnancies, you and your partner can have intercourse and engage in most other sexual activity without harming her or the baby. You and your partner still find each other attractive—if not all the time or in the same ways as before.

However, as the pregnancy progresses, you may have to introduce more variety than you're used to. After all, you have to account for that growing baby bump and all the other changes in your partner's body.

Alternatives Are Fun

The key to sex during your partner's pregnancy is getting creative and trying some things you may not have tried before. There are many ways to connect with each other physically and sexually. If intercourse is too painful or problematic, consider oral sex, masturbation, and creative foreplay for pleasure and intimacy.

Attention, Please

You and your partner can find enormous connection, comfort, and satisfaction in snuggling together, hugging, kissing, saying how much you love each other, massaging, and even talking about your feelings!

However, one alternative sexual activity is off-limits: anal sex. First of all, bacteria from the anus can spread to the vagina and endanger the baby's health. Second, many women develop hemorrhoids during pregnancy (see Chapter 5), making anal sex extremely painful.

On a more positive note, many pregnant women feel freed from the enormous cultural pressure to obsess over their physical appearance. From a very early age, girls and women absorb the idea that they should base their worth on how they look, how much they weigh, and the approval of others. Pregnancy provides a chance for your partner to toss those concerns aside, at least for a while. She can be more in touch with the miracle of how her body works (in this case, growing another human inside of her) than worry about how her body looks. That can lead to a more relaxed, confident, and fun sexual partner for you!

Discovering New Positions

Those changes in your partner's pregnant body mean you have to adjust the ways you have intercourse. This will require both of you to practice, be patient, and experiment. The goal is to use intimacy to bring you together—without causing pain.

As her belly grows, you'll have to abandon the traditional "missionary" position of the man on top and the woman on the bottom. As with many things in life, a simple switch can work.

If you've never tried intercourse with you on the bottom and your partner on top, this is a good time to discover its pleasures. For example, if she has long hair, this method lets her hair play across your face, which can be fun and arousing. Having her on top also gives you easier access to her breasts, which are already likely to become aroused more easily during her pregnancy. Simply lay on your back in bed and help support your partner's body as she lowers herself onto you. This will require patience and adjustments, especially as she gets bigger. You have to maneuver to keep your balance and stability by managing the weight, angles, and positions of your bodies. Instead of the bed, you can try sitting on a (sturdy) chair. This may require still more experimentation as she lowers herself onto you, but it can be worth the effort. If this takes some trial and error, don't worry—that's normal. Don't be afraid to laugh if the maneuvering feels a bit absurd sometimes. Shared laughter can be a great form of intimacy!

Moving back to the bed, many pregnant couples choose the "spoon" position. For this, your partner lies on her side in a semi-curled pose while you lie down behind her, following the curve of her body. This is a very comforting way to cuddle together, snuggling and chatting—even without intercourse. As the saying goes, "Girls like that." In addition, the "spoon" puts you in position for intercourse, entering her vagina from behind. The "spoon" doesn't allow for deep penetration, but it still brings you both pleasure, especially since her clitoris is engorged. And deep penetration is too painful for her as the baby grows and the uterus starts pressuring the lower parts of her torso.

Whatever position you decide on, make sure to pay special attention to your partner's comfort. Because pregnancy hormones loosen up a woman's ligaments and joints so she'll have more flexibility to carry the growing baby and then deliver him, your partner must exert extra effort continuously—and often unconsciously—to hold herself together. (This in one time when "holding myself together" isn't a metaphor!) This work is uncomfortable and tiring. Many women have a lot of back pain as the pregnancy proceeds, which can make intercourse problematic for her. Remain tuned in to her body changes and be willing to go with the flow as you try different sexual activities and positions.

After all, going with the flow may bring new or more intense sexual pleasure for you both. As I mentioned earlier, many women have more orgasms (or have orgasms for the first time) during pregnancy.

A woman's orgasm releases hormones and other chemicals in her body. These "happy" happenings help her relax and feel great—which will, in turn, help the baby feel great. Plus, if sexual relations are part of your continually growing relationship, that's great for the baby, too.

Additional Intimacies

The good news is that intercourse is not the only way to express or experience intimacy. During this time of big transition, it's important to use all of your intimacy tools.

As you already know, your life is undergoing big changes now and will go through even bigger ones once your child is born. Change is stressful, of course, so it's completely natural to seek comfort during times like this.

The best source of comfort for you is your partner, and vice versa. This is a time to embrace affection and physical touch with each other. I'm not talking foreplay, but agenda-free expressions of love, caring, and concern. When you two hug, snuggle, kiss, talk quietly together, and share other physical touch, you show that you value your partner as a whole person—and as your companion on the journey of becoming parents. Affection can bring you to deeper levels of emotional, spiritual, and physical intimacy.

Some expectant couples still struggle with loving physical touch, though. Mood swings tend to be more pronounced for both of you, so one of you may be in an affectionate mood when the other one isn't. At these times, be patient and consistent. Show her random acts of love (such as holding hands, hugging, expressing gratitude, or sharing a smile) that don't always have "let's go to bed" as their ultimate goal. This may take practice, if you've had a pattern of affection always leading to sex. It may not be easy to get away from that pattern, but developing communication beyond physical intimacy is worth the effort. It gives you multiple ways to show that you value each other as much more than sexual mates.

Pregnant Pause

Don't choose the dangerous and shortsighted path of searching for comfort from another sexual relationship. Bumps in the road in your current relationship only get bigger if you chase an emotional or physical affair with someone else.

Being trustworthy is essential for your relationship with your partner—and your child. Violating the sacred trust of those relationships damages your family and you, even if no one ever "catches" you in the act. Think long-term and be the father who understands that your choices influence your children forever.

Listening to the Doctor

Health problems related to sex are uncommon, but some women can face pregnancy risks from intercourse. For example, in rare cases, sex can increase the chances of a miscarriage. Intercourse can also be a risk if you have an active sexually transmitted disease (STD). Remember, the baby has to come through her vagina while it's operating as the birth canal. If there's an STD there, the baby may be infected during birth. While successful sex during pregnancy will take some adjusting in order for you two to find comfortable forms of intimacy, remember that her health (and the baby's) are a higher priority.

The doctor should know if intercourse causes your partner a lot of pain, ongoing cramps, or vaginal bleeding. This is common sense, but sometimes men's judgment gets a little clouded when it comes to sex. Follow the doctor's recommendations—and ask questions if you don't understand her directions fully.

If the doctor explains that certain sexual activity threatens the health of your partner and baby, listen closely. Then, even if it's difficult for you, follow the doctor's suggestions. Your commitment to your baby (and your partner) is more important than a temporary inconvenience.

By the way, there's no need to be shy around the doctor; OB/GYNs and midwives have seen it all (you'll learn more about the doctors you'll be working with in Chapter 7). You're extremely unlikely to convey a concern, ask a question, or discuss a symptom that they haven't heard before. Experience means they won't be embarrassed, so you don't have to be either. Your medical professionals are your resources, so make use of them. Tell them what's on your mind, and keep the conversation going until you have—and understand—the information you need.

You also need to encourage your partner's honesty as you work to find a safe and healthy way to be intimate. She may feel she'll disappoint you if she admits to feeling pain or having cramps. Assure her that you want to know if she's experiencing problems—and that you both have an obligation to communicate those problems to the doctor. Along the way, stay tuned to her needs, while continuing to show affection and other signs of your love for her.

Sex After Childbirth

Your partner's body has been through a marathon by the time she completes pregnancy, labor, and delivery. Nature also has a slew of hormones racing around in her body to help her recover from the delivery and feed the infant.

Even if she's a good athlete in great shape, her body still needs to adjust before she returns to "top-of-her-game" intimacy. She may need her doctor (usually the OB/GYN) to sign off before you two can return to your traditional intercourse patterns.

Your partner's physical recovery from delivery or an episiotomy (see Chapter 12) may make her tired, while leaving her vagina too sore or dry for intercourse. If that's the case, rely on the alternative intimacies you developed during pregnancy until her body and hormones regain their balance.

In addition, both of you will be drained by caring for a newborn 24/7. Maybe one or both of you may be afraid of getting pregnant again so soon after the intense pregnancy, labor, delivery, and infant care scenario.

Pregnant Pause

If you both want to have more children, be sure to discuss how soon you want them. Having that conversation while exhausted from infant care may not be best, but do what works for you.

Don't create a mental calendar for the return of your "old" sex life after your baby arrives. Expectations can set you both up for frustration; the better strategy is to go with the flow—which may lead to "new" things you like better than before you got pregnant. Practice patience and flexibility in your postbirth sex life. Rest assured, these problems don't have to be permanent.

In the meantime, you will have in your hands the incredible baby you created together. Many couples find that miracle of birth and parenthood draws them closer together and enriches their sex life immensely. That's just one way your newborn will provide plenty of joy, love, and valuable distraction.

The Least You Need to Know

- Have fun experimenting with sexual positions and activities before and after childbirth.
- Patience and alternative forms of sexual intimacy will strengthen your relationship with your partner.
- Follow her doctor's guidance on sex to avoid problems.

PART 2

The Pregnancy Path

With a bit of knowledge, you can imagine what's happening inside your partner's belly during pregnancy. Those thoughts can help you start bonding with your baby (or babies) long before she arrives.

However, you're likely to spend just as much time (if not more) concentrating on your partner and trying to cope with the host of changes going on with her. Many of those changes are (or will be) unpredictable. I cover the challenges you'll face in this part.

In this part, you also learn about the intense and wild growth ride the baby takes from egg to exit and get an idea of what to expect during visits to the obstetrician. In other words, this part of the book will prepare you for the next few months—and help you understand why your partner (and you) are also on a wild ride, physically and emotionally.

The First Trimester

In This Chapter

- Your baby, your partner, and you in months 1 through 3
- Coping with hormones
- Helping your partner through the physical and emotional obstacles
- Telling others the news

Determining the exact progression of your partner's pregnancy is an inexact science. Doctors can't really know with certainty the moment of conception, so there isn't a firm date from which to start counting forward. In addition, different embryos and fetuses develop at slightly different rates.

Nevertheless, your partner's pregnancy is already affecting you and her in big ways during the first trimester. She's undergoing physical changes, and both of you will start dealing with psychological, relationship, financial, and other questions. In this chapter, I take you through the first three months of your partner's pregnancy.

What Your Baby's Doing

By about one month after conception, scientists begin to detect a head on the embryo, with a primitive brain and spinal cord.

The brain grows rapidly over the next nine months and beyond. However, it always retains a bit of the primitive, which makes your child's life interesting! Also by the end of the first month, the lungs begin their earliest development and the heartbeat starts.

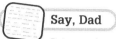

Say, Dad

It is much easier to become a father than to be one.

—Kent Nerburn, author

In the second month, the pace picks up as the embryo grows organs that will eventually turn into eyes, legs, liver, arms, elbows, and facial features. The embryo starts to move, but the limbs are so tiny that their movement is imperceptible to your partner.

If you could climb inside the womb with a microscope during the third month, you'd see the embryo's intestines growing—but on the outside, since there isn't room for them inside yet. You'd also see asexual genitalia and the beginnings of a facial profile. By the end of the month, your child transitions from embryo to fetus because all the major organs are getting in place.

Mom Support

As an "expectant" father, you can't see your baby-to-be until delivery, so there isn't much concrete, observable phenomena to hang your hat on. However, you can see your partner, and she has more than enough observable phenomena to keep you hopping. And compared to what's going on in your partner's uterus, what's going on with her emotions and thought process has a greater impact on your daily life.

Some women have meltdown crying jags every day in the third month, while others have them during the eighth month. Some women have them in both months (and every month in between), and others never have any. There's no surefire "normal" pattern to what a woman will feel as she progresses through pregnancy, nor is there one paint-by-numbers way for a man to experience his partner's pregnancy.

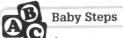 **Baby Steps**

As soon as you find out you're expecting, seek out veteran dads. An experienced father can answer a question (even if it strikes you as a bit silly) because he's probably asked, felt, or thought the same thing himself. Find a man you can share your anxiety, excitement, panic, pride, and uncertainty with. You'll be amazed how much better you'll feel, how much smarter you'll be, and how much more competent you'll be with your partner.

As the expectant dad, you're in a better position than anyone else to make this time satisfying and even fun for both of you. You're also in the best place to help pregnancy deepen your relationship with your partner and your new child. That requires some awareness and work. And the first trimester is the ideal time to begin learning to provide the support your partner needs.

Stopping Alcohol and Drugs

One of the most important changes that needs to be made beginning in the first trimester is stopping alcohol and illicit drug intake.

Your partner should not drink alcohol or use any tobacco or illicit drugs during her pregnancy. When it comes to a pregnant woman drinking alcohol, it enters the placenta and then the fetus. This can permanently damage the fetal brain structure, stunt the baby's growth, and lead to lifelong physical and behavior problems. And smoking while pregnant increases the chances of miscarriage, low birth weight, and infant death. Smoking after the child is born greatly increases the likelihood that she'll develop asthma and other serious breathing problems.

It's very hard for anyone to give up smoking and to break abusive or addictive use of alcohol and other drugs. If your partner has to make these hard choices, it's going to be many times more difficult if you continue smoking, drinking, or using drugs.

If you or your partner resist the idea of giving up alcohol, tobacco, or other drugs, even though they endanger your child's health, that may be a sign you have problem with chemical dependency or addiction. This is certainly not a pleasant thing to consider. The intensity of your resistance may also signal trouble, since denial is a symptom of all addictions.

There's good news, however. Millions of people have recovered (and continue to recover) from chemical dependency, and millions more still struggle with it. If you or your partner have problems staying away from alcohol and drugs, you're not alone.

Look in the phonebook or online for alcohol or drug treatment resources in your area. Or contact these organizations for free information:

- Alcoholics Anonymous: aa.org

- Centers for Disease Control information on tobacco: cdc. gov/tobacco/quit_smoking/index.htm

- Narcotics Anonymous: na.org

- National Institute on Alcohol Abuse and Alcoholism: pubs. niaaa.nih.gov/publications/DrinkingPregnancy_HTML/ pregnancy.htm

- National Organization on Fetal Alcohol Syndrome: nofas. org

- Substance Abuse and Mental Health Services Administration: samhsa.gov

You can also find many tobacco cessation programs through your health-insurance company and your state.

Addictions don't just threaten the fetus or your partner's pregnancy; they also threaten—and often destroy—lives and families. If you suspect that you or your partner have a problem, get it checked out. If necessary, seek treatment and ongoing help so you can both stay clean and sober. It can be an invaluable plus for your child's health and well-being—and can make your family's life a lot healthier and happier.

Moods for Two

Your partner may not know she's pregnant for most (if not all) of the first month. Once she does find out, she'll probably feel bursts of general excitement and anxiety. The feelings may be more intense in her than in you because all of the physical changes she is anticipating in and to her body. She may also be a bit cranky; if her mood gets touchy before getting her period each month, this will look familiar.

Emotionally, the tangible evidence of her pregnancy (such as morning sickness) can accelerate her wide and fluctuating range of feelings.

Meanwhile, your feelings of excitement, anxiety, and so on may not be as intense as hers right now. Why not? Many expectant dads say that in the early months, "the pregnancy didn't seem as real to me as it did to her." In fact, pregnancy is a more "abstract" concept for you during the first month or two, because you can't even see any physical change in her yet.

The second month usually brings the first tests of your patience. She's getting harder to predict, and you have to accept that fact while also doing your best to notice the cues she's giving about how she's feeling. Practice your patience. It's like a muscle that gets stronger with exercise. You'll need that muscle a lot over the next couple of decades!

You may also start having mood swings and bouts of crankiness yourself this month. It's normal to charge back and forth between euphoria and the blues. If feelings of depression hang on without letup for either of you, however, see your doctor for guidance.

Nutrition for Three

Food is a key factor in a pregnant woman's life, and the development of the fetus. However, your partner's choices may not always look logical to you. For instance, she may start having unusual food cravings. (My wife had been a vegetarian for years and suddenly craved steak during her pregnancy.) The key thing is making sure to get your partner the necessary nutrition, because she is now eating for two.

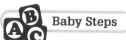 **Baby Steps**

Unless the doctor objects, go along with your part-ner's food cravings. They may change rapidly; something she craved last week may spark nausea today.

You can lead the nutrition initiative by making sure both of you are eating healthy, balanced meals with a full menu of nutrition and vitamins (including folic acid, which can help prevent birth defects). Your partner's digestion may be giving her fits, too, with nausea, constipation, gas, bloating, and heartburn. Keep her as comfortable as you possibly can.

Don't leave all the chores in your partner's hands. You can and should take concrete responsibilities during this time. For example:

- As her body starts to grow out of her clothes, go shopping with her to pick out relaxed, easy-to-use, and easy-to-wash outfits.

- Work to make sure you both are completely avoiding dangerous substances like alcohol, tobacco, illicit drugs, pesticides, and so on.

- Review the medications she takes (even over-the-counter ones) with her doctor.

Throwing yourself into the daily factors of pregnancy gets you in the groove for taking care of your infant, so it's worth the effort!

Wear and Tear

As her body adjusts to pregnancy, your partner may feel physically tired. She may get sleepy more easily, have headaches, or even get dizzy or faint (especially if she has trouble keeping food down).

After three or four months, your partner may be tired of the changes in her body, but she also may have moments of calm about the pregnancy. She also may be urinating more frequently due to her growing uterus starting to pressure her bladder (it'll get worse as the uterus gets really big).

As she becomes more visibly pregnant, the reality of fatherhood may start closing in on you. This can trigger more rounds of emotional reactions (perhaps more intense than previously) of joy and fear from you. You may also feel sexually frustrated; the nausea and vomiting she's feeling aren't very romantic, so you may have trouble getting on the same sexual schedule, or any at all.

 Say, Dad

There are two kinds of people in the world: givers and takers. The takers may eat better, but the givers sleep better.

—Danny Thomas, actor and philanthropist

Keep talking and listening to your partner. If it starts to feel like you're riding a roller coaster, remember how thrilling a real roller coaster is, and that each dip comes before a hill.

Once the bump is starting to show, keep telling her how beautiful she is, because she's probably starting to have that special glow (and because she needs to hear you say it).

What to Expect from the Doctor

If there are no major problems in the pregnancy during her first trimester, your partner will probably have between two and four visits with the doctor. You will need to be at these prenatal visits because this is your pregnancy, too.

At the doctor, your partner can expect to do the following:

- Have a physical to get a baseline for her overall health.

- Give a health history to check for past illnesses and genetic tendencies. Many doctors (wisely) take a health history from the expectant father, too.

- Have blood tests to test for plasma protein-A and human chorionic gonadotropin, which may indicate Down syndrome in the baby.

* Have a urine test to check for kidney or bladder infection, diabetes, dehydration, and preeclampsia (a condition producing high blood pressure and other problems).

* Get a pelvic exam, so the doctor can see the condition of her cervix, ovaries, and other organs.

* Get a pap smear to screen for infections and sexually transmitted diseases. Antibiotics can treat gonorrhea or chlamydia.

At around 12 weeks, most pregnant women will get their first ultrasound (also known as a sonogram). An ultrasound will produce valuable pictures of the fetus, which the doctor uses to check for overall growth, organ development, and potential problems.

Ultrasound technology bounces sound waves off internal organs to capture an image. It's the same basic principle as using radio waves to get a radar image. A technician lubricates your partner's abdomen and then moves a "wand" across her stomach. The wand generates the sound waves, and you can see the results on a monitor.

Fortunately, you walk away with photographic images—and in some cases, video—of your child. Afterward, you'll have a blast showing off the images to everyone you meet.

Pregnancy as a Blueprint for Your Baby

This pregnancy starts messing with your partner's body even before she starts "showing." At different points, she will be irritable, moody, unpredictable, and wonderful. She'll feel nauseous or be unable to get to sleep. Or she won't get enough food to eat and time to sleep. Or she'll burst with enthusiasm, take on new projects, and seem unusually horny for you. Other times, she'll be too exhausted to brush her own teeth. By her third trimester, she'll be big, achy, tired of being pregnant, and peeing every few minutes because the baby is crushing her bladder.

Attention, Please

I wrote much of this book in a coffee shop. One day, a pregnant woman and I just struck up a conversation about my topic. I asked her what she'd tell an expectant father. She said:

"My husband is the subject of all my wrath when I'm pregnant. I can't help myself, and I'm always lashing out at him. Then there are times when I can't keep my hands off him; he seems so sexy and I want him! My advice? Don't take the wrath personally."

Sounds almost completely unpredictable, doesn't it?

Now stop for a moment and shift your focus from living with a pregnant woman to living with a newborn. What does an infant spend time doing?

- Getting irritated, with nothing more than a variation in her cry to tell you why

- Gurgling and giggling when she lays eyes on you

- Peeing (and pooping) over and over and over

- Responding instantly to the feel and smell of your skin and hair by relaxing every muscle in her body

- Getting up in the middle of the night, every night

- Eating on a schedule that defies any order and logic

- Sleeping, waking up, sleeping, and waking up again

As you can see, the course of your partner's pregnancy will mimic the experience of caring for your newborn baby.

Think of pregnancy as a draft blueprint for parenting an infant. Of course, this knowledge might send you into a panic, making you throw up your hands and flee. Take a deep breath—and take comfort in knowing that being an expectant dad gives you some concrete preparation for fathering your child.

Hormone Heaven

Human reproduction is impossible without hormones. Once a couple conceives, hormones have a field day in the woman's body—for the rest of her pregnancy and beyond. You also may experience some hormonal changes as you prepare to become a father.

FSH, hCG, and Friends

Your partner's ovaries have hundreds of thousands of follicles, each containing an unfertilized egg. Follicle-stimulating hormone (FSH) helps the follicles grow and produce estrogen. Estrogen stimulates the lining of the uterus to thicken before ovulation—when the egg starts its monthly journey. A pituitary gland then sends a surge of luteinizing hormones (LH), which triggers ovulation itself. Other cells in the follicle then start producing increased amounts of estrogen and progesterone, which prepare the uterus lining (a.k.a. endometrium) to nurture the implantation of a fertilized egg.

If no sperm reaches the egg, it won't fertilize, and eventually a woman's uterus sheds the endometrium (with hormonal help), resulting in menstruation. However, in a successful conception, the egg has been fertilized, so it attaches to the uterine wall. Your partner is now growing a baby!

Early in pregnancy, your partner's body produces human chorionic gonadotropin (say that three times fast—or even once), known by doctors as hCG, which can be detected in the urine within two weeks of conception. This hormone's cells create the placenta, which also attaches to the wall of the uterus so that it can feed the baby from embryo stage through birth.

A large majority of pregnant women have their hCG levels double every two to three days early in their pregnancy. The acceleration slows a bit by the end of the first trimester, when the levels stabilize until the baby arrives. The surge in hCG may give your partner cramps, nausea, and the need to urinate more often.

Attention, Please

The actual amount of hCG varies from woman to woman, so don't get hung up on the numbers. However, if your partner is getting fertility treatments, the doctor will monitor the hCG levels more closely to make sure they are in the appropriate range.

Progesterone levels also continue to increase during the early months. One of the functions of progesterone during pregnancy is to expand your partner's lung capacity so she can get oxygen to the baby. In the first trimester, this can result in your partner being short of breath.

In the first trimester, pregnancy hormones increase your partner's blood supply, which is essential for your baby's growth. This can affect her nasal membranes, giving her a runny nose, congestion, or nosebleeds. These symptoms usually fade by the end of the first trimester. To help her cope with these issues, encourage her to drink more fluids, consider using a humidifier, and make sure to practice the right techniques to stop a nosebleed.

And while the uterus is hard at work, your partner's hormones are beginning to relax the muscles she uses to digest food during this trimester. For many women, this results in gas buildup—which leads to farting, burping, bloating, and general feelings of discomfort. One way to ease the pain is for her to eat more slowly and eat smaller amounts more frequently during the day; if she goes that route, join her so she doesn't feel left out. Relief can also come from skipping soda, chewing gum, hard candy, and other things that tend to let in more air while eating and drinking.

Elevated hormone levels tend to make pregnant women tired. No surprise, since she's growing a little human in there and her body is preparing to push the baby out. Of course, the emotional and psychological adjustments in anticipating childbirth can bring stress, which usually increases fatigue. If you're concerned about excess exhaustion, talk to the doctor.

Another hormonal issue that your partner may encounter during the early stages of pregnancy is some form of anemia. That means your partner isn't producing enough iron to make sufficient hemoglobin—the part of blood that carries oxygen. Depending on its severity, anemia can bring dizziness, fatigue, weakness, shortness of breath, pale skin, and an irregular or rapid heartbeat. Doctors usually recommend iron supplements to all pregnant women to help prevent or mitigate anemia. You can also urge her to take breaks, avoid stress (if possible), nap, get moderate exercise, and drink fluids.

Finally, pregnancy hormones tend to inhibit hair loss (hers, not yours, unfortunately). Hence, you may notice her hair getting thicker during the first trimester and staying that way for several months after the baby is born. Run your fingers through it to check!

You Have Hormones, Too

Nature finds ways to get a man's attention when his partner is pregnant. Cortisol—the "fight or flight" hormone—tends to rise markedly about a month after a man learns of the pregnancy. No, this is not an excuse to flee; rather, nature is waking you up and heightening your awareness of the big change coming into your life. Increased cortisol levels can also help motivate you to prepare your surroundings for the baby (like the ones I'll discuss in Chapter 8).

As the pregnancy progresses, your levels of testosterone will drop. Rather than making you "less of a man," this hormone change supports a desire to remain close to home and expand into an incredible new dimension of manhood: caring for your child as an involved father.

So why do your hormones change when your body has no baby inside to nourish during pregnancy or breastfeed after birth? Researchers haven't yet discovered a precise scientific answer—and some puzzles remain. For example, *your* level of prolactin—the hormone that triggers lactation in women—rises slightly during *her* pregnancy. Why? That's a stumper, but there you are.

It is clear, however, that your hormone changes seem aimed at getting you ready to be a dad. Take the studies of expectant fathers in the weeks before their child is born, which show they are already better able to hear and respond to an infant's crying than other men who are not fathers. Just know that it's normal to start feeling differently after you find out your partner is pregnant.

And don't scoff at people who talk to you about "sympathy pains," or sympathetic pregnancy. Many expectant dads do feel some of the same physical and psychological symptoms of their partners, known by doctors as Couvade syndrome.

 Attention, Please

Nineteenth-century English anthropologist Sir Edward Burnett Tylor first used the term *Couvade* to identify pregnancy rituals practiced by men in various cultures. Tylor drew it from the French verb *couver,* meaning "brooding" or "hatching."

You may be in perfectly fine health but start to feel nauseous, out of breath, or anxious when your partner is pregnant. This doesn't mean you're sick with a physical or mental problem. Instead, it's probably nature's way of building empathy and connection (emotional and physical) with your baby and her mother.

Couvade symptoms take many forms, don't last forever, and tend to be most noticeable during the first and last trimesters. Other things you may feel include the following:

- Cramps
- Toothaches
- Disruption of your sleeping patterns
- A drop in sex drive
- Changes in appetite
- Depression
- Bloating (really!)
- Backaches
- Restlessness

In most cases, the symptoms are nothing to worry about. In fact, it can be kind of fun to share some of your partner's discomfort—and laugh with her about Couvade's absurd side. Of course, if you're concerned about any symptoms, or if they don't pass, talk to your doctor.

Morning Sickness All Day

It's a rare—and lucky—woman who completes her first trimester without so-called "morning sickness." Despite the name, morning sickness can happen any time of day or night. Most pregnant women have nausea, and about a third will have episodes of vomiting. Some women have nausea and vomiting throughout pregnancy, but it passes for most by the third or fourth month. Unless severe vomiting continues, morning sickness doesn't harm the baby.

The cause of morning sickness isn't entirely clear. One theory holds that morning sickness developed over time as a way for the pregnant mother to repel contaminants that could harm an embryo. Because the embryo hasn't yet developed enzymes that adult bodies use to defend against plant toxins, a pregnant woman's nausea at the sight, smell, or taste of certain foods may be her body protecting the embryo. However, doctors say a woman gifted with no nausea is not at risk for pregnancy problems.

 Baby Steps

You and your partner might find some relief by learning more about theories on the function of morning sickness at mayoclinic.com/health/ nausea-during-pregnancy/AN02133.

Nausea and morning sickness during pregnancy is an age-old issue, so many "remedies" have developed. Keep these suggestions handy when giving whatever support and comfort you can to your partner:

- Try giving her Saltines, dry toast, broth, or gelatin, especially when she's waking up.

- Make sure she eats smaller meals and snacks lightly before going to bed at night.

- Take her to get fresh air—outside and inside your home— to chase away odors.

- Have her try acupuncture or acupressure, which can reduce or relive nausea symptoms.

- Don't smoke around her or let her be near people who smoke.

- Give her ginger ale, ginger tea, or ginger candy. She may not like the taste, but ginger does tend to calm nausea.

- Help her find healthy foods high in protein and complex carbs to eat.

- Make sure she takes her prenatal vitamins faithfully, so her body and the baby's get what they need.

- Consult the doctor about medication for morning sickness.

- Stay positive!

None of the options is foolproof for all women. In addition, some may work for a while and then stop being effective, at which point you have to try others.

If there's no improvement, she's vomiting more than three times a day, she can't keep any food down, or she loses 2 pounds or more, call the doctor. If she vomits blood or dark brown or black material that looks like coffee grounds, get medical care immediately—these can be signs of a stomach rupture.

These problems can be tiring and difficult to be around, especially when your partner is moody. However, it's a lot more difficult for her, so hang in there and support her.

Communication Camp

In case you haven't noticed already, pregnancy is a time of heightened emotion and stress for both of you. The rapid and profound changes can strain your relationship with each other while at the same time drawing you closer together.

It can also be a time of change in your relationship with your family, your career, and the rest of your world. You may worry about how your parents, friends, bosses, and others react to the news. You may be anxious about money, housing, and your future. The best way to handle this kind of change and stress is open and honest communication with people important to you, beginning in this trimester.

You're Both Expecting

When you find out that you're becoming a father, start living by the mantra: communicate, communicate, communicate. Make sure you listen to your partner, encourage her excitement, and understand her anxiety. You should also listen closely to your own body and inner life—after all, one of your most important relationships is the one with yourself.

When it comes to discussing the change in both your lives, avoid asking yes-or-no questions—and giving yes-or-no answers. Open-ended questions give you both a much better chance to learn what the other person is thinking, experiencing, worried about, and excited about. As boys and young men, many of us got little or no coaching in this method of communication. It may take some practice for you now, so be patient with yourself and your partner. Ask for her patience, too.

At its best, having a baby together is a sign of mutual love between the parents. To get the most from your process of becoming an expectant father and new dad, you need to make it a "we" thing. You and your partner made this baby together. When you stop to think about it, that's really a miracle! Therefore, you both should do all you can to make sure you share the experience and what it means.

 Say, Dad

The heart of a father is the masterpiece of nature.

—Antoine François Prévost, eighteenth-century priest and novelist

Start with how you describe the pregnancy and your child. For instance, say, "*We*'re having *our* baby." Seem like a minor point? Well, it's not. When you say "She's having my baby," it sounds like you own both the baby and your partner—a sentiment that may very well make your partner want to scream.

Phrases like "We're having a baby," "We're expecting," or "We're pregnant" tell other people to expect that you will be a full participant in raising this child who's committed to being involved and responsible. This sort of verbiage also helps you and your partner make clear that you won't be shunted aside (or skulk away) when it comes to decisions about the pregnancy and arrival of this new child.

The other thing you should be sure to say to your partner is "you're beautiful" and "I love you." Often. Most days, these words will come quite easily. Many expectant fathers (myself included) report that their partners seemed to glow during pregnancy. And having a baby might well be the most intimate thing two people can do together. Other days, when hormones and energy (yours and hers both) are riding the Tilt-A-Whirl, you may need every ounce of discipline to tell her that she's beautiful and lovable. Do it anyway.

Don't fall prey to "second banana" jealousy. Yes, other people may put the spotlight on your partner when they talk about or react to the pregnancy. Nevertheless, you have the capacity to prevent other people's attitudes from diminishing your connection to your partner and your newborn. You and your partner are more important to the baby than anyone else; use that knowledge to keep your perspective.

On the practical front, start screening health-care professionals for your pregnancy and delivery. Go to the doctor with your partner and facilitate communication by advocating for her and making sure that the health-care professionals hear and answer questions from both of you (more on this in Chapter 7).

When to Tell the Rest of the World

You and your partner are the only ones who get to decide when and how to tell people your good news. Some expectant parents wait until after their first ultrasound, when they know more about any fetal risks and the rate of miscarriage drops—though keeping a problem pregnancy a secret might make it harder to get the support needed later on. Other parents reveal the news earlier because they're eager to share the excitement. Either way is just fine!

Be considerate of people's feelings, especially any sense of feeling left out. With the first few people you tell (parents, siblings, and close friends), consider telling them to keep the news a secret until you give the green light. This reduces the odds that a loved one is offended because "you told *her* before you told me?!" And be prudent with your use of social media to tell everyone about your baby. You're asking for trouble if news of your impending fatherhood reaches your parents first on Facebook.

The method you use to deliver the news should fit your own style. Some people print up matching "we're pregnant" T-shirts or buttons. Some mark cards from a sonogram image, or wrap up the news in a present and record reaction on video (for example, making a YouTube video). Enjoy the moment however you share it!

The Word at Work

When it comes to the office, be smart about breaking the news. It's better to present the news directly and in context, as opposed to thinking of the pregnancy as some ill-timed event (like a death) you need to "break" to someone. And tell your boss before you tell Twitter. You don't have to hide your excitement, but you also need to put yourself in your boss's shoes. (I'll give you more detail on planning your work life in Chapter 9.)

 Attention, Please

According to the U.S. Equal Employment Opportunity Commission, federal law forbids discrimination against a woman based on pregnancy when it comes to any aspect of employment, including hiring and firing. The picture is much less clear for the "pregnant" father. Rare states (for example, California) mandate parental leave for dads and moms. Check the laws in your state to see what they say about paternity and maternity leave.

Anticipate the boss's questions about the pregnancy, the due date, and other issues, especially your plans for taking time off. Your manager needs to plan for changes in the workforce, so the more prep time, the better. If you want to explore or negotiate any lasting changes in your responsibilities or schedule—to deal with problems during the pregnancy or to clear space to actively raise your child— ask the boss if you can set a time for you two to discuss the options. After all, your job and financial security are important to your soon-to-be-growing family.

The Least You Need to Know

- Make sure you're a constant support to your partner during the first trimester, as she begins to go through many physical and emotional changes.

- You're also changing—for good reasons—as you begin to prepare to become a father.

- You can set the tone and set the limits when spreading the news of the pregnancy.

- Be smart and strategic when you communicate with your partner and others about the baby during this early time of dramatic adjustment.

The Second Trimester

In This Chapter

- Keeping your partner comfortable
- Taking childbirth classes
- Preparing for multiples
- Learning CPR and other first aid for your baby

By the second trimester of your partner's pregnancy, things start to feel more concrete and real. As her body grows, so does your awareness that you'll indeed become a father soon. You're lucky that pregnancy takes nine months, so you have time to adjust "gradually" to the enormous changes soon to enter your life.

In this chapter, I tell you about different kinds of childbirth classes, what you can do to help your partner with some common pregnancy discomforts, and what happens when you have more than one baby. Don't worry, you can survive all of these things!

What Your Baby's Doing

During the middle months of pregnancy, your baby's development continues to speed forward. In the fourth month, his growing body makes room to house the intestines, and they will then move inside the growing body. The fetus also begins to develop vocal chords and starts growing his fingernails, swallowing, and urinating. A doctor may even be able to detect a heartbeat using a fetal monitor.

In month five, the fetus starts moving his eyes slowly and can begin coordinating the movement of his ever-growing limbs. Girls start developing ovaries (with enough eggs to repeat this whole process some years down the road). Toenails also begin to appear at this time. The head is still much larger than the rest of the body, but the difference is narrowing.

By the beginning of month six, many mothers can feel "quickening," a vague sense that something's moving in there. Some women say it's like air or a water balloon inside them. Boys will develop testes and girls their vagina and uterus. The fetus may start hiccupping and will grow eyebrows, along with other fine body hair. Some expectant moms can also perceive distinct movement by the end of six months.

Mom Support

As pregnancy marches on, your partner will face new challenges. As usual, your support will help her through. Keep encouraging healthy eating and physical activity for both of you. And if her energy or commitment flag, demonstrate a burst of enthusiasm to help her out. But remember: you won't be perfect, and you don't need to be.

Here are a few difficulties you need to understand (and help out with) to help her through the second trimester and beyond.

Relieving Leg Cramps

Your partner's body is getting larger and working overtime to nurture a second person. This puts new stress on her legs and feet, which commonly results in leg cramps. While the cause is unknown, these cramps usually happen at night during a pregnancy's last six months.

Here are a few simple ways you can help your partner prevent leg cramps:

- Make sure she drinks water and sports drinks. If you're an athlete, you know that hydration helps with cramps—and overall health, too.

- Keep her physically active; movement keeps the muscles more resilient. However, as she gets larger, consult with the doctor for an appropriate exercise routine.

- Advise her to wear smart shoes. At this point, high heels are pointless—and unhelpful. Recommend shoes with strong heel support and lots of comfort; utility must trump fashion now.

- Buy magnesium supplements or foods high in magnesium for her, as consuming it can help prevent leg cramps. Nuts, seeds, beans, whole grains, and dried fruit are good sources of magnesium. Your partner should check with the doctor before starting a magnesium supplement. (Some prenatal vitamin preparations include magnesium already.)

- Help her remember to stretch her muscles and join in yourself—all you need is a wall and a floor. Stretching is always smart, especially right before going to sleep.

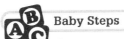 **Baby Steps**

If your partner would like to learn some stretches to help her avoid leg cramps, have her check out the "How to Stretch a Calf Cramp" video (youtu.be/VUYf-Nqkf2k).

If a leg cramp comes, it will probably arrive with little or no warning. Don't ask her for an explanation; just ask her "Which side?" Massage the muscle (using ice, if that helps) or hold the ball of her foot while you gently push it upward to stretch out the muscle fibers and relieve the pain. After the initial spasms, she may still be sore. A warm bath, hot shower, or ice pack can help with any of the residual soreness.

Treating and Preventing Hemorrhoids

The larger the fetus gets, the more weight presses down on the organs in your partner's lower torso. This can strain her vascular system and give her constipation, both of which lead to hemorrhoids—swollen, inflamed veins inside the anus or under the skin around the anus. In addition, her veins may be more prone to swell because hormones can relax the vein walls during pregnancy. If your partner also stands or sits for hours each day, the added pressure on her veins can cause them to swell into hemorrhoids.

Hemorrhoids (also known as piles) have a bad reputation for good reason. They can be very painful and itchy, especially when trying to pass a bowel movement.

Because hemorrhoids are most likely during the third trimester (when the baby is heaviest), it's best to work on preventing them now, in the second trimester. You can't keep the baby from pressing down on her veins, but you can take steps to reduce the other hemorrhoid culprit: constipation.

The following are ways you can help your partner avoid hemorrhoids:

* Make sure she drinks plenty of water, at least eight glasses' worth every day.

* Serve her raw fruit, raw vegetables, and other high-fiber food; the fiber cuts down on gas.

* Exercise with her at a moderate pace (again, following the doctor's recommendations).

- Recommend that she use the toilet as soon the urge hits; waiting even a short time increases the pain and difficulty of making a bowel movement.

- If she sits a lot (for example, at work), encourage her to stand up and move around regularly. This keeps the digestive system more flexible and temporarily lessens the pressure of baby's weight.

Fortunately, hemorrhoids usually go away on their own. In the meantime, she can find relief by taking a sitz bath or soaking her rectum in warm water for 15 minutes several times a day (one more way pregnancy can be quite time consuming). She can also use an ice pack to reduce the swelling.

Talk to the doctor for other options; anything you can do to prevent, shorten, and relive the discomfort is a huge plus. If your partner has rectal bleeding, get to a doctor. You need to make sure the bleeding is not from something a more serious than hemorrhoids.

Adjusting Seat Belts

Traveling gets more complicated as your partner's belly grows. One of the changes is how the seat belt lies on your partner. For best use, it's important to help her adjust the seat belt to fit properly and protect her and the baby.

 Pregnant Pause

It's a myth that seat belts and airbags are dangerous for pregnant women. They are by far the best protection for her and the baby in an accident.

Keep the following things in mind when adjusting your partner's seat belt:

- Adjust the belt so it lies across her pelvis (or what remains of her hips), below the belly. Do *not* place the lap part of the belt above or over her belly.

- Pass the shoulder part of the belt between her breasts, not near her neck.

- Do *not* put the shoulder belt behind her back or under her arm. The shoulder strap may not be super comfortable above her belly and across her chest, but that's where it belongs.

- Keep the air bags on, but do *not* use them as substitutes for seat belts. The two technologies work in tandem to protect you both during a collision.

Driving can get tricky as your partner's abdomen grows, especially if she's short. The U.S. National Highway Traffic Safety Administration (nhtsa.gov) recommends that a pregnant woman keep her breastbone at least 10 inches back from the steering wheel (when she's driving) or dashboard (when she's a passenger). As she expands, move the seat back so her belly is clear of the steering wheel—but not so far that her feet can't reach the pedals easily. If, eventually, she can't do both, someone else (most likely, you) will need to drive.

Cleaning House

If you're like a lot of couples, your partner does most of the housework. Now is the perfect time to change that dynamic. Pregnancy is frequently making her achy and taxing her energy, so step up your Mr. Clean game as the pregnancy progresses—and stick with it after childbirth.

The modern world doesn't have many work tasks that you can thoroughly complete; that's one of the things that makes housework so satisfying. Once you dust and vacuum a room, it's clean. Sure, it'll need cleaning again in a couple of weeks, but right now, you have closure and pride in finishing an entire task in a relatively short period of time.

If the notion of cleaning a toilet grosses you out, this is the best time to get over it. Starting in a few months (and for the following couple of years), you'll be handling poop daily. It won't be your own and it won't be dropping neatly into a toilet. Once the baby is here, cleaning the john might become a nice reprieve from changing diapers, so get the hang of it now.

If at all possible, do a complete and comprehensive scouring of your home. Once the baby moves in, neither you nor your partner will have much time available for dusting, vacuuming, and cleaning the toilet. So seize the moment (and the mop) now!

What to Expect from the Doctor

Second-trimester doctor visits happen about once a month. The doctor will check your partner's blood pressure and weight while also measuring her abdomen to assess the baby's growth. She'll also check the fetal heartbeat (and probably let you hear it, too).

Your partner will also have at least one ultrasound during the second trimester. The primary purpose is to check for any problems, but by now the doctor can also tell whether you're having more than one baby and tell the gender of your baby/babies.

The doctor will also take blood and urine samples from your partner to check for the following:

* Infections (such as yeast infections, sinusitis, bronchitis, and the like)

* Anemia

* Gestational diabetes

* The level of four pregnancy hormones, which can signal if she needs further testing for potential birth defects

An important test the doctor may do at this time is to see if your partner has Rh-negative blood. Rh is a protein on red blood cells, which carry oxygen throughout the body. Most people have the protein (and are Rh-positive), but others don't (and are, therefore, Rh-negative).

If a pregnant woman is Rh-negative and her fetus is Rh-positive, there can be problems. The baby's blood can cross over into the mother's bloodstream, where her body treats the Rh protein as a foreign substance and creates antibodies to fight it. However, if those antibodies travel into the placenta, they can also attack the *baby's* red blood cells, destroying them faster than they can be replaced. This serious condition, called *hemolytic anemia,* can keep the baby from getting enough oxygen.

Fortunately, there is effective treatment if the problem is recognized in time. Injections of Rh immune globulin can keep your partner's body from making the potentially dangerous antibodies. You can see why doctors are so diligent in screening for Rh incompatibility.

As with all other visits, bring along any questions or concerns and make sure you get complete and comprehensible answers.

Childbirth Classes

By the second trimester, you need to start taking childbirth classes with your partner so you both learn—and practice—your roles during labor and delivery. If you want to be a real partner in childbirth and childrearing, your attendance is a non-negotiable must.

You and your partner can choose from a number of different (but related) and reputable approaches, but they all emphasize two crucial points:

- Pregnancy and childbirth are natural processes, not diseases that need to be cured.

- As coach, friend, and partner, you are your partner's most crucial resource in pregnancy, labor, and delivery.

Hospitals, birthing centers, and some community agencies offer childbirth classes, often with sliding-fee scales. They're an essential investment of your time and money, so make sure you participate. Get the dates, times, and location of each class and cement them in your calendar.

The Lamaze Method

The most widespread childbirth classes relay on the Lamaze method (lamaze.org). Created by Dr. Ferdinand Lamaze of France in the 1950s, this method teaches relaxation, external focus, and breathing techniques to manage pain and to help parents ease the journey through labor and delivery. This method stresses that childbirth is a natural process and therefore should be treated that way, and that babies shouldn't be separated from their mothers at birth. The goal of the Lamaze method is avoiding anesthetics when giving birth, although a birth is still natural even if your partner needs pain-killing drugs (see Chapter 11).

You're central to the Lamaze method. You coach and do the concentration techniques, relaxation exercises, and breathing exercises with your partner during the pregnancy (for practice) and during labor and delivery (for the real thing). And because Lamaze encourages the mother to move around during labor and focus on relieving discomfort, you're her primary calm and comfort resource. Lamaze childbirth class will provide you with some tactics to help her relax, such as massage, ice chips, and more.

When taking Lamaze classes with your partner, you'll probably see videos about labor and delivery. If you think these videos will gross or creep you out, use your viewing as a constructive desensitization experience to reduce the chance that you freak out in the delivery room. You also get information on caesarean deliveries, epidurals, and the like.

 Attention, Please

Many childbirth education organizations have videos, online classes, mentors, and other support you can access through the web. Check their websites for the latest resources.

The Bradley Method

The Bradley method (bradleybirth.com), touted by The American Academy of Husband-Coached Childbirth, emphasizes healthy nutrition, being an informed consumer of medical services, and the active involvement of fathers. Bradley also wants parents to be in charge of both the arrangements for labor and delivery and what happens during those times, while also being prepared for emergency interventions (such as caesareans). This method is named for Robert Bradley, a Kansas obstetrician who started lobbying in the 1940s to get husbands into the delivery room. It focuses on the whole length of the pregnancy and the early months of life.

The Bradley method tends to have more weeks of class than the Lamaze method, but it also covers a wider range of topics. Bradley relies on breathing and relaxation. Like Lamaze, it also encourages the mother's focus to be internal, rather than external. With the Bradley method, your partner learns how to close her eyes and get in tune with what's happening inside her body, with the goal of smoothing the process and reducing pain. The expectant father is key to coaching the mother through this process and keeping her focused.

Also like Lamaze, Bradley classes teach you how to support your partner during labor, such as through coaching her breathing, working with her to relax, and being an advocate for the both of you with the hospital and professionals. You also learn how to massage the baby after birth.

Leboyer

Leboyer is the name often used for two approaches using water to ease the newborn's transition from the womb to the world. During the 1970s, French obstetrician Frederick Leboyer experimented with making birth rooms more womblike, because he thought the bright lights, noise, and activity of the "normal" hospital delivery room was too much of a shock for a baby emerging from the dark, muffled, warm, and liquid environment of the uterus. To replicate the uterus, he called for immersing the newborn into a small tub of warm water (called a "Leboyer bath") and giving him a massage right away. He also argued that the baby should stay on the mother's stomach for bonding rather than being rushed away for examination and testing.

Some people also use the term *Leboyer* to describe the practice of having the mother and father partially submerged in warm water for labor and delivery, using a tub specially designed for that purpose. The baby is born underwater and then placed on the mother's abdomen or at her breast for some time before cutting the umbilical cord. Michel Odent, a Leboyer follower, popularized this method. Although there isn't an official Leboyer organization, you can learn more about the water-based approach at the Waterbirth International website: waterbirth.org.

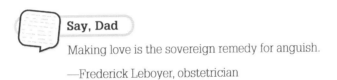

Say, Dad

Making love is the sovereign remedy for anguish.

—Frederick Leboyer, obstetrician

Both approaches are not only meant to reduce the shock and stress of birth for the baby; they also benefit for parents. The calm, warm surroundings can also cut down on parents' anxiety as the baby is born.

Some research supports the Leboyer approaches to childbirth, showing that babies born into dark, quiet rooms are calmer and more alert than other newborns. Some hospitals have even installed birthing pools and created quieter labor and delivery rooms to support these approaches, but check to be sure they have the expertise to use them at maximum potential.

HypnoBirthing

HypnoBirthing (hypnobirthing.com) teaches women to self-hypnotize and use slow breathing methods that move in concert with her contractions. The theory is that removing fear and tension will naturally lead to less pain.

Ideally, hypnosis helps a woman moderate or even eliminate labor pain while increasing a relaxed state of concentration. Certified hypnotherapist Marie Mongan pioneered HypnoBirthing and says the idea is "to actually relax the woman's body to the point it can work the way it was designed to work."

During HypnoBirthing, the father helps the mother with breathing, performs light massage to keep her relaxed and focused, and is the main point of contact between her and midwives and doctors. During HypnoBirthing classes, you and your partner practice "scripts" for relaxation and maintaining a calm mental state for both of you. You also learn ways to help condition your partner's mind to relax and respond to your prompts, assuring her that she can deliver the baby.

Birthing From Within

Birthing From Within (birthingfromwithin.com) approaches pregnancy and childbirth as a rite of passage. Think of it as another strategy for staying mindful and relaxed in the moments and hours of labor and delivery. Birthing From Within advocates a focus on the mother and father doing the best they can, without being committed to a specific outcome (such as no drugs, no cesarean, and so on).

The goal of Birthing From Within is not getting too hung up on "controlling" the birth; instead, it's about using self-awareness and relaxation to let things happen as they happen. Obviously, both you and your partner have to buy into this approach (or any approach, for that matter) in order for it to be effective.

The BirthingFrom Within model offers classes on early pregnancy, childbirth preparation, postpartum connections, and healing from a cesarean.

The Payoff

By going to childbirth classes and learning effective coaching techniques, you help your partner (and you) feel and be more in control of the pregnancy, labor, and delivery. The more you know, the more you can decide what works for you during the whole birth process.

Because you've taken these classes, you'll be able to guide, encourage, and comfort your partner as you two go through a stressful and miraculous time together. During labor, nothing beats your hands massaging her limbs, your fingers placing an ice chip between her lips, or your loving voice telling her that she can do this. Best of all, being the coach means you'll get to be there in person to witness your own child entering the world. Nearly every father who talks about being at his child's birth describes it as an incredible high and a miraculous experience.

 Say, Dad

A nurse snapped a couple of photographs as I held my newborn twins for the first time. In every shot, I look awestruck—because I was.

—Asante, father

And don't overlook another excellent reason to be a birth coach: connecting with other dads. At childbirth classes, you'll meet other men who are expecting (most for the first time) just like you. In a good childbirth class, you'll have at least one session that includes a presentation from a veteran father about what to expect. If the class you take doesn't feature this, speak up and say you want it. Because I saw firsthand in Lamaze classes that other men were interested in (and even excited about) being intimately involved in their partners' pregnancies, I felt comfortable making conversation and comparing notes with other expectant fathers in the OB ward while my wife was in labor. Plus, your life as a father will be more satisfying (and easier) if you keep up these relationships with other dads after you leave the hospital. For me personally, it's like carrying the Lamaze intensity I learned into all the rest of my fatherhood.

If you'd like more information about childbirth, check out these other resources for expectant parents:

- The Association of Labor Assistants and Childbirth Educators: alace.org

- Childbirth and Postpartum Professional Association: cappa.net

- International Childbirth Education Association: icea.org

Preparing for Bonus Babies

Most pregnancies conclude with the birth of one healthy baby. On occasion, however, you might find another baby (or two or three) in there.

In North America, an ultrasound usually detects multiple fetuses by the middle of a pregnancy. It wasn't always that way. As recently as the early 1980s, doctors didn't use ultrasounds as a matter of course—they reserved it for women showing indications of trouble with trouble pregnancies.

Routine ultrasounds eliminate that level of drama for most couples today ... but it's still exciting on those rare occasions when the doctor delivers a baby, only to shout, "Wait a minute; there's another one in there!"

The rate of multiple births (in other words, a pregnancy producing more than one child) is rising in the United States, in part because more people are using fertility treatments to get pregnant (see Chapter 2).

The most common multiple is twins. Fraternal twins can be two girls, two boys, or one of each. The term "fraternal" refers to the fact that these infants are no different than siblings born years apart; each child has a unique genetic makeup. That's because they come from two different fertilized eggs inside a mom. Identical twins come from a single fertilized egg that splits early in pregnancy. That means identical twins have identical genetic codes; they are humanity's only genuine clones. Thus, you get only one gender: two boys or two girls. You also have kids who look exactly alike—although they may (or may not) have very divergent personalities.

From 1980 to 2010, the number of twins born in the United States more than doubled, and the number of triplets more than quadrupled. Women over 30 are naturally more likely than younger women to have a multiple birth, and more over-30 women are getting pregnant than a generation or two ago, leading to this increase. In addition, improvements in infertility treatments mean that more women use fertility strategies to get pregnant. Because fertility treatments stimulate the release of eggs from the follicles, they also increase the odds that more than one egg will be fertilized—and more than one baby born.

 Attention, Please

According to the Census Bureau, of the nearly four million live births in the United States during 2010, about 3.6 percent were multiples. Of those, 5,503 were triplets, 313 were quadruplets, and only 37 were quintuplets or more.

If you have more than two babies, doctors call that "higher-order multiples." You will soon be correcting the doctors, explaining that the more accurate way to describe raising triplets or quadruplets is "higher-order chaos." Triplets, quadruplets, and quintuplets are much rarer than twin births. You're most likely to see a higher-order multiple birth among older women and women who take fertility drugs—but they're still unusual.

Whether there are two, three, or more, multiple fetuses take up a lot of room in a uterus, giving them extra incentive to exit early. Therefore, many multiples are born prematurely or by caesarian. Due to medical advances, far more multiples survive childbirth and infancy than ever before.

And because they have to share their mother's nutrition during pregnancy (and be born prematurely), twins and other multiples are often physically smaller than a singleton (twin slang for babies born solo). Many remain smaller all their lives, and sometimes one twin is smaller than the other. A multiple may fall behind singletons in development of language skills, although that usually doesn't reflect on their intelligence.

Attention, Please

The best central resource for parents of multiples has an unfortunate name, in the context of a book for fathers-to-be. The National Organization of Mothers of Twins Clubs (nomotc.org) has excellent tips, resources, and support. They also have local chapters called, more appropriately, "Parents of Multiples Clubs."

If you find out you're having multiples, you need to ask for and accept the help and kindness of friends and family. Fortunately, other people frequently come forward to lend a hand—and an extra crib or car seat. I experienced this as the parent of newborn twins, and nearly every other "multiple" parent I know met the same generosity.

Having multiples also means you need to prepare to make a radical adjustment in your schedule, because no parent can manage more than one infant alone—not for more than a few hours, anyway. The most practical result of discovering multiples via ultrasound may be the weeks and months you get to adjust your work life. Don't wait to make parenting, daycare, career, parental leave, and other arrangements before the babies arrive (see Part 3 for more about this preparation).

Infant CPR and First Aid

Along with your other preparation and education, consider learning how to perform cardio-pulmonary resuscitation (CPR) on an infant and other essential first aid at this time, while you have a few months to go. You're unlikely to ever encounter such a crisis with your baby, but it helps to be prepared. Knowing these skills can also help someone else's child in an emergency.

You can take an infant CPR training class through your local Red Cross chapter, hospital, fire department, or emergency medical services agency. The procedure isn't complicated, but it's markedly different than CPR you'd perform on an adult. Usually running about four hours, the class gives "hand-on" training and practice to help you stay calm and confident if you ever have to put your skill to work. You can also download a simplified Red Cross explanation of infant CPR, resuscitation for a baby who has stopped breathing, and ways to respond to choking at redcross.org/images/MEDIA_ CustomProductCatalog/m4240175_Pediatric_ready_reference.pdf.

You can watch online videos or purchase DVDs from the American Academy of Pediatrics or the American Heart Association, but they won't be as comprehensive as an in-person raining. If you'd like to supplement your training, you can watch a good, short overview video featuring Cleveland Clinic and Red Cross experts at health. discovery.com/tv-shows/baby-week/videos/baby-health-infant-cpr. htm.

You should also assemble a first aid kit for the baby. The kit can include the following:

* Ipecac syrup (to induce vomiting if the baby swallows certain toxins)

* Infant acetaminophen; it comes in liquid form and usually includes a medicine dropper with measurements. (Never give an infant adult acetaminophen or aspirin.)

* Baby nail clippers

* Cotton balls (Don't use cotton swabs to clean the baby's nose or ears.)

* Baby thermometer

* Bulb syringe/nasal aspirator

* Antibiotic cream

* Sterile gauze

* Baby gas drops (a.k.a. simethicone)

* Disinfecting hand soap (for you)

* Baby wash cloths and wipes

The contents are simple, so consider having one at home, in your vehicles, and other places the baby will be regularly. You can also purchase a fully assembled infant first aid kit, although that will be more expensive.

Remember, whenever you have an emergency with your baby (or anyone else), one of your first moves should be to call 911. They will dispatch skilled emergency medical technicians (EMTs) or trained police officers to help.

The Least You Need to Know

- Help your wife through some of the common issues in the second trimester, such as leg cramps and adjusting the seat belt to fit her pregnant belly.
- Your participation in childbirth classes is essential and a great way to get in touch with other expectant dads.
- You can enjoy "multiples" with preparation and the willingness to ask for help from family and friends.
- Infant CPR and first aid training can ease your mind and provide you skills to help your baby in an emergency.

The Third Trimester

In This Chapter

- Managing your partner's body
- Watching for trouble signs
- Dealing with delays
- The worst-case scenarios: miscarriage and infant death

Emotionally, the third trimester can bring a roller coaster of anticipation and agitation as childbirth and the challenges of mothering draws closer. Some pregnant women get quite calm, some get a bit more anxious, some become very excited, some are downright impatient, and others swing around through a number of moods.

Try re-reading the previous paragraph and substituting "expectant dads" for "pregnant women." Good, now you know how you're going to feel, too.

In this chapter, I discuss the changes and challenges that occur during the third trimester of pregnancy.

What Your Baby's Doing

In month seven, the fetus' hearing has improved to the point that she can hear her mother's organs at work (how scientists know this is beyond me, but they do). The growth of her brain also really takes off during this time. And the lungs, while still not nearly developed, have grown enough so that the fetus could survive (with tons of medical attention) if she were born.

Depending on a host of factors, the fetus reaches the point of viability in the seventh or eighth month, meaning she can live outside of the uterus. As you might imagine, each day of growth *inside* the uterus improves your baby's chance for viability and reduces ongoing health problems.

 Attention, Please

The baby may feel simultaneously more real and more mysterious for you in the waning days of pregnancy. Remember that those feelings are not contradictory; a new baby is real *and* a mystery, which is part of what makes her so wonderful and fun.

During the eighth month, the fetus's eyes are open, with eyelids to help, and she may begin to suck her thumb. Fat is building up under her skin, and she can surpass 5 pounds in weight (if she's in there alone). She may start having predictable sleep patterns. However, when awake, she will be moving so much that you should have no trouble feeling (and maybe seeing) the movement on your partner's belly. She may now be able to distinguish different sounds, including your voice (so talk to her!).

By the ninth month, the baby is (ideally) head down in the uterus, and plumb out of space. With no room to kick, she'll wiggle and squirm instead. Brain growth continues at warp speed, packing on more fat and weight, and by the end of the month, she may "drop" down into your partner's pelvis in preparation to leave (which puts lots of pressure on your partner's bladder). Her fingernails have already grown full length, so she may start to scratch herself. (It often seems that boys continue scratching themselves for the rest of their lives, but in utero, girls do it, too.)

Mom Support

Your visits to the doctor are more frequent during the last trimester, as the doctor keeps a close eye out for potential complications that can affect labor and delivery. Your partner is dealing not only with her ballooned body, but also the potential of being put on bed rest.

First, recognize how well your partner is handling all this, and that will reassure you she'll be fine. You can then use your concern about your partner's well-being as motivation for a positive attitude about any issues that crop up during the last trimester—and continue to maintain your routine of healthy eating, exercising, and getting your lives ready for your baby.

A Whale of a Woman

Your partner is coming down the home stretch with a heavy load. This is probably causing major aches in her back, pelvis, legs, and feet. The growing baby inside also makes it harder to maneuver her body through what used to be simple daily activities.

Her center of gravity shifts from her backside (normal for everyone) to her abdomen and breasts. She may feel (and often be) less graceful and have to figure out new habits for doing simple things with so much baby in the way. For example, my daughter works as a barista. She's short, so she must lean forward quite a way over the sinks to reach the faucets. But by the time she was eight months pregnant, her belly was so big that I couldn't use the sink anymore!

In addition to making her huge on the outside, your partner's growing uterus is crowding her other organs like someone with a huge backpack on a subway car at rush hour. One set of organs being squeezed is her lungs, meaning she has to concentrate a bit more on breathing. Not to worry, though; the baby still gets plenty of oxygen—after all, nature has been at this birthing thing for a long time.

Once the baby "drops" (shifts down into the pelvic area in the days/weeks before birth), she may have less difficulty breathing, but she's liable to feel slightly different stresses on her back and legs. The baby has run out of room to move around in there, so she's probably feeling more squirming and less kicking. By your partner's due date, she's as huge as she's going to get, with many physical discomforts.

If your partner describes herself as a whale as these changes happen, she has that right. After all, she's a lot bigger than she's used to being. You, on the other hand, should avoid using the term anywhere she can hear it—or within earshot of anyone who has any chance of ever speaking to your partner at any time in the future.

Instead, support her through the physical and emotional challenges of her size at this stage. For example, her altered body proportions increase the chances that she'll lose her balance. So help her maneuver safely around the house. Also, provide comfort at the times she's overwhelmed by the new obstacles brought about by her pregnant body.

The Pregnancy Detective

During this time, it may be hard to tell if your pregnant partner is being overly stoic or has become a raging hypochondriac. In some ways, hypochondria may be the better approach right now. Here's why: illnesses which don't cause major concern at other times of life (like the flu) can become quite risky when a woman is pregnant.

With your doctor's support, you can keep an eye out for symptoms and clues that may indicate a problem. This is especially important if your partner doesn't notice (or doesn't admit) when she gets sick.

To help get you started, here are a few illnesses and infections that she may (or, if you're lucky, may not) encounter while pregnant:

The flu is unpleasant to get anytime, but especially during pregnancy. Influenza increases the risk of severe illness for your partner while also raising the chance of serious problems for your baby, including premature labor and delivery. The best way to prevent this is both you and your partner getting a flu shot. Flu shots are safe for pregnant women and (because influenza is contagious) a smart investment for you, too. If your partner develops symptoms—fever, chills, aches (more than she already has), diarrhea, vomiting, sore throat, and so on—call the doctor right away.

Milder flulike symptoms may come from an infection called *toxo-plasmosis*. It's caused by a parasite found in raw (or undercooked) meat, dirt, and cat feces. Toxoplasmosis can cause serious health problems for the baby (such as blindness or mental disability), so the doctor should be checking for it. You can help your partner avoid getting toxoplasmosis by washing all produce, cooking meat thoroughly, and making sure you both wash hands and utensils after touching raw meat or soil. And absolutely do not let her clean the cat's litter box. (Sorry, man, that's your job for the duration.)

Urinary tract infection (UTI) is exactly what it sounds like. Symptoms include burning while urinating; pelvis, side, back, and stomach pain; chills; fever; shaking; and the sweats. If the infection spreads to the kidneys, it can trigger premature labor and damage your partner's health. Talk to the doctor if she's showing signs of a UTI; the doctor will probably prescribe an antibiotic.

 Pregnant Pause

A substantial number of women struggle with eating disorders (binge eating disorder, compulsive overeating, anorexia, bulimia, and related problems). They pose a serious danger at any point in a person's life, but the danger is magnified during pregnancy and childbirth. If your partner shows signs of an eating disorder, she needs immediate help from a psychologist, physician, or nutritionist well-versed in these complex disorders. Above all, don't try to solve this problem on your own. You can read more about anorexia and bulimia and pregnancy at nationaleatingdisorders.org/pregnancy-and-eating-disorders. You can read about binge eating disorder and pregnancy at bingeeatingtherapy.com/2011/11/18/friday-qa-pregnant-stop-binge-eating/.

Yeast infections result when the natural yeast in your partner's vagina goes into overdrive—a common problem during pregnancy. The baby is in no danger, but your partner will be very uncomfortable with vaginal itch, swelling, burning, and discharge. Yeast infections can usually be treated with over-the-counter antifungal creams or suppositories without harming the baby. Consult your doctor.

Like yeast infections, *bacterial vaginosis* results from too much "natural" bacteria in the vagina. Symptoms include burning and itching while urinating and a foul-smelling grey or white discharge. Bacterial vaginosis may contribute to low birth weight or premature birth. If your partner has this, the doctor will treat it with an antibiotic.

Diabetes and *gestational diabetes* threaten the fetus *and* the mother. In gestational diabetes, your partner's blood sugar is too high, increasing the risk for premature birth, C-section, and (ironically) low blood sugar in the baby, among other problems. The doctor should screen your partner for the gestational variety, regardless of her medical history. If she already had type 1 or type 2 diabetes before getting pregnant, make sure the doctor and the rest of the health team know it. If she has either of these, the doctor will look to control her blood sugar via meal plans or prescriptions. Whatever the doctor orders, help your partner stick to it for the safety of her and your baby.

Be sure to ask the doctor what else you can do to stay alert for signs of problems in the pregnancy. You are around your partner much more often than the doctor, so your observations can be a great resource.

Anything But Bed Rest!

Bed rest doesn't "cure" problems in pregnancy, but it can reduce or slow them down. A doctor may order it at any time during pregnancy, although it tends to be more likely in the last month or two. Common reasons for bed rest include the following:

- A cervix that's dilating early or is "incompetent," meaning it's likely to dilate too soon

- A multiple-baby pregnancy

- Problems with the placenta or the baby's growth

- Vaginal bleeding

- Indications that the woman may go into premature labor

Pregnant Pause

Many pregnant women want to keep working as long as possible before the baby comes. Sometimes, that desire can go a bit overboard. For example, in the summer of 2013, Silicon Valley executive Carl Guardino was meeting on the phone with a colleague. Soon, he could tell that she seemed out of breath. Guardino told the *San Jose Mercury News,* "I asked if she was all right, and she said, 'Actually, I'm at the hospital. And I'm in labor.'" Wisely, he proposed that they end the call and meet some other time!

Bed rest has various levels of intensity. The doctor may simply instruct your partner to ease up on her workload or spend less time on her feet. At the other extreme, she might be admitted to a hospital because the problems are severe or bed rest at home hasn't done the trick.

So what do you do if the doctor tells your partner she needs complete bed rest? First, hope your partner isn't running huge projects at work. Second, pray that she can live without her job and its income while enjoying relaxed (or is it bored?) days and weeks flat on her back or side. No matter the situation, you have to be the enforcer.

My wife was on strict home bed rest because her cervix had started dilating a month early (because we were having twins, although we didn't know that yet). A Type-A store manager, she claims she kept firmly to her bed for the few days before her water broke (and bed rest became moot). My recollection? She got up much more often than I thought necessary or prudent.

It doesn't matter which one of our memories is correct. It does matter that you realize how difficult and stressful bed rest can be for both of you. Use all the coaching and encouragement you can to keep her horizontal! The following are some things you can do to help:

- Make her health and bed rest your first priority. The baby's health (and hers) depend on it, so put other things on the back burner for the time being.

- Bring meals, snacks, and drinks to her in bed.

- If you're not home for some meals, prepare them ahead of time and store them in a cooler she can reach from bed. If there's room, put a microwave on a side table so she can heat up food, make popcorn, and so on.

- Have entertainment (books, computer/tablet, audio, and TV) within easy reach.

- Arrange for visitors to come. This breaks up the day and provides good distraction for her.

- Spend lots of time with her when you're home, since she'd likely to be spinning her wheels alone when you're out.

- Call in reinforcements. Ask relatives and friends to take a shift, make a meal, lend a movie, and so on so you have periodic breaks.

- Keep her comfortable. Arrange pillows, chairs, and other furniture to minimize aches, pains, and irritation.

- Remind her to stay in bed!

- Stay upbeat, especially if the bed rest drags on for days and weeks.

Yes, she may well go bat crazy—and you may be tempted to follow along. But remember the big picture: this situation is temporary, and it's helping your baby be born in the best condition possible. Someday, you'll laugh about this (really!) and wonder if either one of you will ever want to have breakfast in bed again.

What to Expect from the Doctor

The doctor will test for a bacteria called Group B strep (GBS) during the third trimester. About 25 percent of women have GBS in their vaginas, even if they're not pregnant. It's rare for GBS to pass from the mother to the baby—or even for the mother to have any problematic symptoms. However, if GBS does infect the baby during delivery, it can produce breathing problems, heart and blood pressure instability, gastrointestinal and kidney problems, sepsis, pneumonia, and meningitis.

The test doesn't hurt; the doctor will swab her vagina and anus and then send the sample off to a lab for testing. If your partner has GBS, she'll get an antibiotic during labor to prevent passing it on to the baby.

Say, Dad

You know your children are growing up when they stop asking you where they came from and refuse to tell you where they're going.

—P. J. O'Rourke, satirist and political humorist

Meanwhile, the doctor will continue to monitor your partner's blood pressure, weight, and other vital signs. Some of these routine tests may require your partner to supply a urine sample. In terms of your baby's health, the doctor will check on the baby's size, movements, and heartbeat.

If this is a high-risk pregnancy (for example, high blood pressure, diabetes, or multiples), your partner may need additional tests designed to see how the baby is responding to any current stress— and how she may respond to the stress of labor itself. These tests may include the following:

- "Targeted" ultrasound, which uses high-frequency waves to get more precise images of the fetus.

- Cervical length measurement, which uses an ultrasound to determine any risk for preterm labor.

- Vaginal secretion tests, which involves swabbing the vagina to screen for levels of fetal fibronectin, the "glue" that holds the sac against the uterine lining.

- Cordocentesis (a.k.a. percutaneous umbilical blood sampling), which looks for infections and chromosome irregularities.

* Fetal heart monitoring combined with ultrasound, to perform a nonstress test of the baby's heart and general well-being.

When the Baby's Late

If your partner's pregnancy enters its tenth month, all parties have probably lost patience. Yes, Papa, there can be a tenth month, although what seems like the tenth month may just be a case of the doctor miscalculating your conception date. Remember that the normal "term" of a pregnancy falls between 38 and 40 weeks from the first day of conception. That's a wide window to begin with, and a baby occasionally stays in there beyond 40 weeks.

Beside which, the due date is always an estimate; despite all the research and books, science still hasn't learned everything there is to know about every single pregnancy. It is known, however, that "overdue" pregnancy is more likely if it's your partner's first pregnancy, you're having a boy, or your partner has problems with obesity.

The keyword at this point is *patience.* Your baby is still growing like a weed (a pattern she'll follow for years after she finally pops out), and she isn't going to stay in there forever.

Meanwhile, your partner is probably going to be battling achiness, hemorrhoids, heartburn, shortness of breath, sleeplessness, and even frustration.

What can you do to help?

* Remind her (and yourself) that this pregnancy really is nearing the end.

* Be skeptical of nonmedical "cures," such as nipple stimulation, herbal remedies, eating spicy food, acupuncture, and having more sex. All of these may be enjoyable or relaxing, but don't expect them to suddenly stimulate labor.

* Encourage gentle exercise, as long as it's comfortable for her. Walking and standing can keep things loose and help tire her out for a better sleep.

- Listen. Your partner is likely to moan and complain about her discomfort. Be sympathetic, and don't take it personally if she says, "Why did you do this to me?" That's the hormones talking (and you'll hear that refrain again once labor starts!).

- Use the "extra" time to stock up on frozen meals, straighten up the house, or go to the movies.

- Keep communicating with the doctor. She'll be checking your partner every week (if not more often) to monitor the fetal heartbeat, check the cervix, and so on.

- Get to those appointments, so you remain in the know and on the same page with everyone else.

- Discuss options (such as inducing labor) with your partner and the doctor. Even if you don't need "alternatives" in the end, talking about them can relieve some of the anxiety of waiting.

Overall, your best bet is to practice acceptance. The situation—and your feelings about it—are what they are. You'll make it through!

Miscarriage and Infant Death

On an intellectual level, you understand that you don't know who your baby will be. At the same time, it's completely normal (and fun) to fantasize about what you plan to do with your baby once she's born.

Unfortunately, some of children die in infancy or never survive in the womb. These are hard realities to acknowledge, and hard realities to live through as an expectant dad.

Miscarriage means the embryo or fetus doesn't survive until birth. Miscarriages are caused by genetics, hormones, serious infections, anatomic abnormalities, and other, rarer issues. In nearly every case, you and your partner can't control these things. Most miscarriages happen early in pregnancy; the chance of miscarriage decreases as the pregnancy progresses. *Infant death* is the death of a child during the first few hours, days, or months after birth.

Nearly all miscarriages, infant deaths, and birth problems happen just by chance. Nothing the parents did or didn't do during pregnancy caused it, and it's not their fault. Literally millions of chemical and biological sequences must happen in the right order for an embryo or fetus to survive pregnancy and an infant to survive the early days of life. Improvements in health care and standard of living have reduced—but probably will never eliminate—miscarriages and infant deaths.

Infant death and miscarriage bring grief to both parents. Unfortunately, many people minimize the expectant father's loss because he never saw the baby. That attitude is gravely mistaken. The baby didn't stir within your uterus, but she was real to you, whether or not she was born.

Cultural attitudes that frown on men being sad—combined with parents' different physical experiences of pregnancy and childbirth—may complicate your own sense of grief. The following sections talk briefly about these painful moments and what you can do to deal with your grief.

End-of-Life Decisions

Preterm and critically ill babies are more likely to survive their birth due to medical advances. For example, babies can be kept alive after as little as 24 weeks in utero, even if they weigh between 1 and 2 pounds. However, these survivors often have major physical and mental issues, like blindness, heart and lung problems, cerebral palsy, and more.

In addition, these babies have the highest risk of infant mortality during their first hours, days, weeks, or months. This means parents (and physicians) may face enormous ethical and emotional decisions about the care an infant gets.

Not surprisingly, research suggests that good communication and trusting relationships between parents and health-care providers will reduce stress on the parents. In addition, effective palliative or hospice care provide essential support for parents and facilitate their decision-making.

Attention Please

Palliative care is a multidisciplinary approach to easing and preventing suffering in sick people. It is used for people with chronic diseases, as well as those nearing death.

Hospice care provides terminally ill people with palliative care while also giving emotional, psychological, social, and spiritual support to the patient and her or his family.

There's no way to describe adequately the challenge of making end-of-life decisions for your own child. If you find yourself in this situation, it is essential that you get a lot of support.

Naomi Tzril Saks, MDiv, is chaplain for the neonatal palliative care team at Kaiser Hospital Oakland. Once the prospect of recovery has passed, Saks says the goal is to give meaning and comfort to the infant and her family during her final days.

Therefore, Saks says, some end-of-life decisions may be influenced by a range of parental desires: "From allowing time for distant family to arrive and performing a baptism to photographing the infant in clothing that has special meaning." Such steps help parents absorb the importance of their relationship with this child, which can then help the grieving process.

Most hospitals with neonatal intensive care units offer some level of palliative care, but it may be harder to find resources for infant hospice care. If you have to cobble together a few resources, go for it. Good hospice care is an amazing gift that can turn an extremely painful situation into a time of comfort, peace, and connection for you, your partner, your child, and your family.

Hiding from Grief

You shouldn't feel any shame if your baby died or was miscarried, because you did nothing wrong. You have every right to grieve. However, you must realize you and your partner may grieve this loss in different ways.

Surviving a miscarriage or child's death is *not* a matter of competing over who is grieving the most. There's no way to compare, even if comparing was the point (which it isn't). It's a matter of understanding how you're expressing your grief, and—since you and your partner are not the same person—understanding that she may very well express hers differently.

Some people think that grief is harder for men than it is for women because men supposedly "hide" their inner feelings. However, I think we men always reveal our feelings but are socialized not to do it directly. This, in turn, causes us to have trouble expressing our feelings in a way that's understandable to others.

Indirect expressions of grief might include burying yourself in your job or house projects, drinking, or marathon TV watching. Such activities can work well as temporary distractions. But restricting yourself to "distraction" behaviors will keep you in isolation and prolong your difficulties. You may also rebel at the thought of joining a support group and get tired of your partner's sadness and want to "move on."

You must find healthy ways to work through your grief directly. No single method works for everyone, so you may need to try a few strategies along your journey. This is perfectly normal under the circumstances. Consider one or more of these approaches:

- Work with an individual therapist or counselor.

- Visit a therapist or counselor with your partner to address how your relationship responds to your loss.

- Talk with your clergy or spiritual advisor.

- Participate in a grief and loss group. One place to start looking is nationalshare.org/Groups.html.

- Use online resources for information and support, such as marchofdimes.com/loss-grief.aspx and babylosscomfort. com.

- Encourage family and friends to learn appropriate ways to support a grieving parent, such as "What to say to a griever" at griefspeaks.com/id6.html and "What *not* to say to a griever" at griefspeaks.com/id9.html.

* Remember that you aren't alone, so don't *be* alone too much. Reach out to other parents who've lost a child. They can't "solve" your problem, but they can understand you.

Attention, Please

Miscarriage and infant death are traumatic events. Some research suggests that symptoms of post-traumatic stress disorder (PTSD) can be found up to 18 years after a miscarriage or infant death. However, parents who used effective support systems fared better than those who didn't.

It's very difficult to deal directly with this trauma and can often be difficult to deal with the path of finding and using support. Nevertheless, a direct approach is still the best, because it brings the best results for you.

Living with Your Loved Ones Afterward

The death of a child after birth or because of a miscarriage can put serious strain on a marriage or relationship. This kind of trauma can draw you and your partner closer, or drive you apart.

Here are some steps to help you grieve and keep your relationship strong:

* Care about each other, your feelings, and your needs, even when that's hard to do.

* Keep an open line of communication to share your thoughts and emotions.

* Accept your differences and acknowledge each other's pain.

* Dedicate yourself to your relationship, and assure your partner of your commitment.

* Talk about your baby and find ways to remember her.

When it comes to friends and other family members, they may have trouble talking about the loss with you and your partner, which can lead to some stupid or insensitive comments or actions. In your desire to comfort yourself, your partner, or your family, you may fall into the same trap. Here are some important things to avoid saying or doing:

- Let your anger or sadness stop you from getting support and love.

- "We can always have another child to replace this one." You may have another child, but there is no "replacement" for this particular child you created together.

- Be afraid to talk openly with your partner, family, and friends about your loss.

- "You/I/we shouldn't feel sad anymore." If you're open (especially with your partner) about your grief and get support, you will move on with your life. However, this loss will always be sad.

- Blame the miscarriage or infant death on yourself or your partner. It wasn't your fault, and there's already enough guilt after such a loss.

- Pretend that this didn't happen to you, or that it's no big deal. Don't let your family and friends pretend this either.

Think of it this way: If your partner or parent died this Friday, no one (including you) would expect you back at work on Monday morning with all your feelings swept away and arrangements tidied up as if nothing had happened. So don't expect something different when you've just lost a child, even one you never saw or held.

Miscarriage and infant death are real losses that bring both you and your partner real grief, anger, frustration, and feelings of helplessness. Respect the loss and honor your baby by taking your grief seriously—and grieving together with your partner as best you can.

The Least You Need to Know

■ Help your partner maneuver her growing and shifting body to increase comfort and reduce the risk of a fall.

■ You can be the doctor's eyes and ears to help detect pregnancy complications.

■ If your partner is put on bed rest, be the enforcer and make sure she relaxes.

■ Keep perspective and practice patience if the pregnancy goes into overtime.

■ Miscarriage and infant death impact both you and your partner. Attend to your grief, anger, and recovery together.

The New Life Plan

Preparation for parenthood isn't all about emotions and relationships. You also have many practical, nitty-gritty details to work out.

Part 3 explains a smart approach to screening and picking the doctor, hospital, and child-care professionals you need to line up in the coming months. You also learn how to keep the professionals listening to both you and your partner.

In this part, I also go through how to prepare your home for the day your baby arrives there for the first time. You learn how to lay out a "nursery" space and how to safely outfit your home and car with must-have gear for infant care.

In addition, you have to prepare your life outside of the home. This part gives you a quick survey of legal and financial issues that come up in regard to your new baby, such as establishing paternity and creating a will. I also give you practical tips on preparing your work life (including your boss and colleagues) for your transition to fatherhood.

Choosing Doctors and Other Professionals

In This Chapter

- Picking your support staff
- Accompanying your partner to appointments
- Keeping your place in the health-care process
- Looking at daycare options

If you're like most men, you've never had any reason to visit a gynecologist. You also probably have no experience finding reliable daycare providers or deciding the merits of a midwife versus an obstetrician. When it comes to pregnancy and birth, you've probably never seen a baby born before, and terms such as "amniocentesis" and "chorionic villus sampling" are most likely not in your regular vocabulary.

This chapter gives you a framework for finding the professionals you and your partner need to achieve a successful birth and infancy for your baby. I also coach you on how to find your place and make your voice heard with these folks.

Finding the Right Medical

Professional

Picking an OB/GYN, CNM, doula, or other professional requires careful thought and consideration. These folks are key players in a successful birth and will be on your mind a lot over the next few months. Therefore, you must be able to communicate and work together.

Some expectant couples are comfortable following the professional's lead—confident that the doctor knows best, they don't feel the need to question her recommendations. They view the doctor as the captain, not a colleague, on the pregnancy voyage. Other couples want a more collegial relationship with their pregnancy professionals. They want to ask many questions, probe the doctor's reasoning, make suggestions, and explore alternatives. After all, the mom will be doing most of the work, with the dad by her side. Why shouldn't both have substantial input?

Each approach is perfectly legitimate, as are any approaches that fall somewhere in the middle. The key is to find someone who's compatible with the plan you and your partner have for the pregnancy and delivery of your baby.

Who to Look For

The first medical professional you can look into is your family practice physician, as some have experience overseeing pregnancies and delivering babies. If you're already comfortable with your family practice physician, that can make the process easier for you and your partner.

One of the most common professionals expectant parents go to is an obstetrician/gynecologist (OB/GYN). Your partner is likely to stick with her current gynecologist if she has one, likes the doctor, and the doctor is an obstetrician. However, not every gynecologist does obstetrics, which involves caring for women and their reproduction organs during pregnancy, labor, delivery, and after the child is born. An OB/GYN also makes sure the fetus is healthy. If you and your partner aren't already connected with an OB/GYN, ACOG has a "Find a Doctor" tool at acog.org/About_ACOG/Find_an_Ob-Gyn.

Another professional who works with expectant parents is a midwife. In the centuries before hospitals, many families relied on midwives to handle labor and delivery. Today, a Certified Nurse Midwife (CNM) has specialized training that isn't restricted to labor and delivery. She (a few midwives are men, but not many) is skilled in low-risk pregnancy, reproductive health, well-woman exams, primary health care, breastfeeding, and other postpartum needs. According to the National Center for Health Statistics, CNMs "attended" (in other words, participated in) 7.8 percent of U.S. births and 11.6 percent of all vaginal births during 2010.

 Attention, Please

CNMs are also trained to recognize signs of problems in your partner's pregnancy, labor, and delivery. If necessary, they can call in the resources of an obstetrics specialist.

A CNM must have a Master's degree in nursing and pass state licensing exams. More than half of CNMs work for a hospital or physician's practice, but they also work in private practices or as part of a birthing center. Medicaid covers CNM services nationwide, but only 33 states require private health insurers to reimburse for a CNM.

Many couples who choose a CNM like the commitment to holistic health and the more relaxed approach to childbirth. Like a good OB/GYN, a CNM will provide education, suggest resources, or refer you to additional health-care providers if needed. A CNM may have more time during an appointment than some busy OB/GYNs to listen to your concerns and address problems. Like ACOG, the American College of Nurse-Midwives has an online tool to help you locate a CNM in your area: midwife.org/rp/find.cfm.

A less well-known pregnancy resource is a doula, whose work also has its roots in ancient midwifery. While not medical professionals, reputable doulas are trained to support a woman through her pregnancy, labor, and delivery. Doulas often participate in home births but are less common in hospital settings.

A doula will meet with you both during the pregnancy, sharing information and coaching you to prepare for childbirth. She'll (male doulas are also rare) strive to build confidence and ease fears for you and your partner, as well as aim for a calm, relaxing labor and delivery atmosphere that facilitates your partner's natural childbirth instincts.

Because there's no "officially recognized" accreditation for doulas, many traditional medical care providers are skeptical of their value. However, a comprehensive University of Toronto study found that pregnant women were less likely to need cesareans and epidurals if they used a midwife or doula and had fewer delivery complications. Of course, this may be due in part to the fact that midwives and doulas usually stick to low-risk pregnancies—still, the findings are interesting.

In a growing number of places in the United States and Canada, OB/GYNs, CNMs, and doulas work together on a professional team to help women through pregnancy, labor, and delivery. This is a bonus for you, since the cooperation reduces conflict and mistrust on your pregnancy support team.

However, what if your partner's pregnancy is more complicated? Depending on your circumstances, she may need referrals to other medical professionals. One possible specialized physician you may have to work with is a perinatologist, an obstetrician who treats women with special medical problems during pregnancy due to her heredity, chronic illnesses, or other factors.

What to Ask

Now that you know about the different professionals you may want or need, how do you choose the right one for you and your partner? Here are a few questions you two can ask to help you find the right person:

* Tell us about your approach to pregnancy, labor, and delivery. For example, how do you decide when or whether to recommend pain drugs or a caesarian section during labor?

* Are you able and willing to deliver the baby in the birthing center or hospital we want to use?

* How many babies have you delivered, and how long have you been doing this?

* Where did you earn your MD and get your OB training?

- Do you have colleagues or former patients willing to give a reference?

- What do you usually recommend for a woman who has gone past her due date?

- Who will handle our labor and delivery if you're not available? Do we have any say in who that will be? Can we meet him or her?

- How will you manage our birth plan? Will all of your colleagues know where to find it—and how to respect it?

- Can we ask questions or send you information via email or text? What's the best way to call you or your office, especially after hours?

- Do you have a midwife or doula on your team? If not, are you willing to work with one?

 Pregnant Pause

You have the right to screen for the professionals who will be part of your team; in fact, reputable OB/GYNs, CNMs, doulas, and other professionals expect potential patients to interview them. Consider it a major red flag if the person you're thinking of bringing on isn't willing to have such a conversation.

Remember, this isn't a final exam for you to grade. These questions are tools to help you find professionals who share—or at least, are willing to work with—your values and plans for pregnancy and childbirth. Don't just disqualify someone if she or he doesn't answer every question exactly as you want; listen to the nonverbal signals and to your gut when talking with a professional. Does she strike you as receptive to and comfortable with the conversation? Can you understand what he's talking about, and is he willing to help if you don't understand?

You don't need to become BFFs with the doctor. However, since you do have to trust and respect her, it helps if you like her, too. Should your partner decide to use her current gynecologist or family practice physician, make sure you meet that doctor as early as possible in the pregnancy. You and the physician need to get a sense of one another and learn how to cooperate.

The ultimate goal is to find someone who you and your partner can work with. You may never see the doctor again after your baby is born, so don't look for a lifelong mutual admiration pact. However, you and your partner should be able to work together with this person during a key period of your life.

Your Hospital Options

Your baby will be born somewhere, so you and your partner need to decide whether to deliver in a hospital, birthing center, or at home.

Hospitals are the most common location for childbirth. Your OB/GYN or CNM will be associated with the labor and delivery department at one or more hospitals, meaning your choice of doctor will affect which hospitals you can consider. Hospitals tend to be large and institutional, with an environment that some people find cold and less personal. However, many hospitals now use designs and practices that borrow from birthing centers (more on them in a minute). A nearby hospital may have birthing tubs, labor or post-birth rooms with a bed for you, facilities for involvement by relatives (including children), and even luxuries like massage and fancy meals.

If your partner is giving birth in a hospital, be sure to visit the facilities beforehand. Nearly all hospital labor and delivery departments offer expectant parents a tour of their units. While there, ask questions and read the vibe to get a sense of how willing they'll be to respect your wishes and include you in the process.

Birthing centers or *birth centers* are homelike facilities near or inside a hospital that are often staffed by CNMs. Birthing centers are usually cheaper than hospitals, and proponents say the birthing center approach cuts down on the number of C-sections.

Birthing center advocates also argue that the childbirth experience can be impeded by the ways hospitals operate. Birthing centers are less likely to have as many staff shift changes, nursing shortages, strict chains of command, and other bureaucracy. Their more relaxed environments can therefore make them more responsive to you and your partner. Birthing centers also tend to be more family friendly than hospitals. For example, there's seldom a problem with other children and relatives being present for labor and delivery.

 Attention, Please

For some laughs related to home birth—and several other aspects of fathering—watch comedian Jim Gaffigan's riff on kids at youtu.be/GEbZrY0G9PI.

According to the National Association of Childbearing Centers, birthing centers use a "wellness" model of pregnancy and birth that emphasizes that childbirth is natural and not a disease. So you won't find major anesthesia at most birthing centers. They rely instead on movement, massage, whirlpools, and other tools to deal with labor pain.

However, a birthing center is still a medical facility, with trained nurses, fetal monitors, infant warmers, and so on. Its staff will draw on a network of specialists if complications arise, and because they are close to hospitals, they can get you and your partner to one quickly if need be. Birthing centers are regulated by states, and accredited by (wait for it) the Commission for the Accreditation of Birth Centers. You can find out more about birthing centers at birthcenters.org.

Home birth means planning to have the baby at home, as opposed to an emergency home delivery (which I'll discuss in Chapter 11). You and your partner may consider home birth because it keeps you all in a familiar and presumably less stressful environment. For example, your partner can have more freedom of movement, use her own shower, eat from her own refrigerator, and so on. Family, cultural, or religious tradition may also influence the decision.

Having a home birth requires working ahead of time with the CNM or doctor who will oversee it to figure out what services will be provided and what will happen if complications arise.

Doctors don't recommend home birth if your partner has health issues, such as diabetes, seizures, high blood pressure, anemia, preterm labor, or other problems. And if she uses tobacco or illegal drugs, a birth at home is too risky. In addition, home birth is usually ruled out if you're having multiples, the baby isn't positioned properly in the birth canal, or if your partner had a previous baby by C-section.

Are You In or Out?

Regardless of whether your partner has had a baby before (and especially if she hasn't), she needs every ounce of moral support you can give her. Going with her to the doctor is tangible support she can see and feel.

You'll find that the vast majority of OB/GYNs, midwives, and hospitals now expect and allow the father to be present for labor and delivery. This is a radical change from 50 years ago, when OB wards only tolerated men in the waiting room.

However, some habits and attitudes in this type of profession die hard. Men still report being ignored, belittled, or barely tolerated when accompanying their partners to obstetrician appointments—and even in labor and delivery rooms. Technicians, secretaries, doctors, or nurses may view you as an annoyance, distraction, or "cute" appendage to your partner's pregnancy. As fathering expert Armin Brott says, "The fact that the dad-to-be might have some specific and important needs, concerns, questions, worries, or anything else of his own rarely seems to occur to anyone."

What do you do if you encounter these attitudes? Basically, you have three options:

- Resent these people and lash out at them.

- Resent these people and brood in silence.

- Find effective ways to speak up for yourself and work with these people.

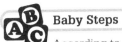 **Baby Steps**

According to 2009 statistics from the American Congress of Obstetricians and Gynecologists (ACOG), 47 percent of OB/GYNs in the United States are women. In 2010, women earned 48 percent of U.S. medical degrees; however, more than 80 percent of medical school residents now specializing in obstetrics are female.

Don't let the gender of the obstetrician be a communication barrier. After all, the level of the doctor's qualities is not a function of gender. So do your best not to judge the ability of your doctor (and other pregnancy and childbirth professionals) by it.

Of course, the last option is most constructive for you, your partner, and your baby. It may feel unfair that you have to be reasonable when someone else is being unreasonable, rigid, or pig-headed. On a certain level, it *is* unfair to be ignored or treated as a distraction in the doctor's office. Nevertheless, as a partner and father, you have bigger challenges right now, and being there for your partner is most important. Besides, learning this kind of patience can help you in the future (just wait until your 2-year-old starts throwing a tantrum!).

To show the doctor and others in the doctor's office you want to be included, you can use some or all of the following strategies with calmness, consistency, and resolve:

- Greet and introduce yourself to every professional you encounter, from the front desk staff to the doctor, at the first appointment and again at the next appointment. Repetition will help them get the point—and remember you.

- Look, act, and be interested in what's going on.

- Engage in the conversations between the doctor and your partner. Don't be aggressive or interrupt your partner, but (literally) make your voice heard.

- Ask questions about both the pregnancy and your own needs and preparation for fatherhood. If the doctor's answers aren't clear or if they leave you with more questions, ask follow-up questions. If the doctor doesn't have answers, ask where you can get them.

- If you're not being included (by the doctor or your partner), don't wait and expect that they'll eventually get around to inviting you—involve yourself.

- Recognize that most "dad isn't important" attitudes result from entrenched bad habits, not personal malevolence toward you.

- Make your physical presence felt. Don't threaten or intimidate anyone, but don't sit in the corner either.

- Demonstrate in your words and actions that you are just as concerned about the well-being of your partner and baby as the doctor is.

If the medical professionals you deal with are particularly obtuse, you and your partner may have to directly and calmly tell them you want—and expect—to be included in the process. You may then have to repeat your message occasionally (although not as often as you will with your 2-year-old). If the doctor or others in the office don't get the message, you and your partner can switch practitioners.

 Say, Dad

My idea of an agreeable person is a person who agrees with me.

—Benjamin Disraeli, writer and British prime minister

The Gynecologist Will See You Now

Some expectant dads dismiss the idea of visiting an OB/GYN's office. What's the point of a man going to a "lady doctor"?

If you don't participate in your partner's OB/GYN appointments, you risk conveying the idea (to you partner, the doctor, and others) that you're dismissive of the pregnancy's importance. As you recall for the previous section, you want to avoid that at all costs. Accompanying your partner to her doctor visits helps set the pattern of you two accompanying each other on the lifelong journey of parenting. So unless you're hospitalized or held hostage somewhere, show up for OB/GYN appointments—especially the first one.

The last, best reason for going to every OB/GYN appointment is how it engages you in the pregnancy. A lot of what's happening in the pregnancy is abstract to the expectant father—or certainly more abstract than to your partner, who's getting her belly kicked from the inside out.

Being part of this world makes things more real for you and helps you prepare psychologically for early fatherhood. You'll be able to hear the baby's heartbeat via the doctor's stethoscope and probably have your first look at the baby as a grainy, swimming image on the doctor's sonogram machine.

But you can't experience any of that if you don't show up. And one of the first rules of fathering is "show up."

Dad's Role on Visits

When you're in the doctor's office, concentrate on doing two things:

* Give your partner the support she needs. Be upbeat and cheer her on.

* Advocate with and for her. If you've been waiting in the examination room for a half hour, be the one who goes and finds out why. Make sure the doctor answers all of her questions—and yours.

That advocacy role can really pay off for you, your partner, and the baby. If your face is familiar to the doctor throughout the pregnancy, then she'll remember your investment when "labor day" rolls around. Human nature tends to help people (even doctors) respond well to other people who respect them and show interest in what they do.

During the first visit, you and your partner will be answering questions. Someone will take a health history from each of you, looking out for current conditions or past diseases that may signal potential problems in pregnancy and childbirth.

Be honest with your answers. For example, you may be embarrassed to reveal that you have a sexually transmitted disease (STD). However, an active STD can pose a serious risk to the baby during delivery. The doctor needs to know this information. Besides, your medical history remains confidential, and unless you have smallpox (the last case was reported in 1977), your past and present illnesses won't surprise an experienced physician.

Before going to an appointment, use a notepad (paper or digital) to write down questions you've gathered (and want answered) before your first appointment or since your last appointment and any information you want to pass along. These can be things like the following:

- Can you suggest more comfortable ways for her to sleep at night?

- Over the last couple weeks, she's been experiencing (*fill in the blank*). Is that normal?

Remember to bring the notebook with you—you'll be amazed how easy it is to leave things behind when rushing to the doctor. Make sure you get satisfactory answers to all of the questions you and your partner have. After all, while your partner's distracted by blood tests and pelvic exams, she might have trouble remembering what she wanted to ask. Don't forget to write down the answers, too, so you don't forget the information when you get back home.

 Attention, Please

Fatherhood might require radical modifications in your own health behavior. Ask the doctor for guidance for improving your own health. If the doctor doesn't know, or doesn't have time to discuss it with you, ask her to recommend another physician who can. Then go see that doctor! Research shows that men are reluctant to seek medical attention until a problem has gotten beyond the point when early intervention works.

Ultrasounds and Finding Out Your Baby's Gender

During each visit, the doctor will monitor the pregnancy's progress, especially with regard to the health of your partner and the baby. In the world of medicine, monitoring health or disease translates into tests. Beyond the home pregnancy kit, the best-known pregnancy test is the ultrasound, known by medicine as obstetric ultrasonography.

This technology sends sound waves through a woman's belly to visualize the baby inside the uterus. The sound waves bounce back to a machine, which interprets them and produces an image of the fetus. As the fetus grows, the ultrasound can pick up more detail.

Around 13 weeks into the pregnancy, an ultrasound can make out the baby's genitals and, thus (in most cases), the baby's sex. Once this information is available, you and your partner have a few options:

* Have the doctor or ultrasound technician tell you if it's a girl or a boy. Share the news with everyone you know ASAP.

* Have the doctor or ultrasound technician to tell you if it's a girl or a boy. Keep the news to yourself (or a small circle of sworn-to-secrecy friends and relatives) until later in the pregnancy or after the baby is born.

* Keep the baby's sex a mystery, even from yourselves, until he's born. Instruct the doctor, ultrasound tech, and other medical professionals you want to be surprised at the moment of birth, so they should keep the information to themselves.

I'm a fan of the last option because I like suspense and have trouble keeping secrets. I also like it because, for eons, people only discovered the baby's sex when he (or they) came out of the mom. Perhaps that makes me a traditionalist?

On the other hand, if the ultrasound machine knows, why shouldn't you know, too? The technology's "early warning" capability still gives you a moment of surprise and excitement. And knowing the baby's sex lets you celebrate a new aspect of the pregnancy with other people (or not), even before the baby arrives.

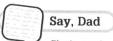

Say, Dad

She's got her looks from her father. He's a plastic surgeon.

—Groucho Marx, comedian and actor

Whatever route you take, take it together. Diverging approaches on this issue invites trouble. Remember how pregnancy mimics your future? There are some important times in parenting that you and your partner need to be on the same page. Whether you and your partner should find out your baby's gender may be the first one.

Here Come the Needles and Gloves

During pregnancy visits, the doctor's staff will always do a few routine tasks, such as checking your partner's weight, blood pressure, heart rate, and other vitals.

The doctor will also take blood and urine samples periodically, and perhaps order some additional tests. Those additional tests may include the following:

- **Amniocenteses:** A procedure in which the doctor inserts a thin, sterilized needle through the woman's abdomen and into the amniotic sac, which holds the baby, to capture a small amount of amniotic fluid. The doctor uses the fluid to test for signs of abnormalities or illness.

- **Chorionic villus sampling (CVS):** A test where the doctor inserts a catheter through the vagina in order to capture a sample of tissue from the placenta. This is used to screen for genetic defects. One advantage of CVS is that it can be done at 10-and-a-half weeks, while amniocenteses must wait until between 17 and 20 weeks.

- **Fetal monitoring:** The doctor will use a stethoscope or, if she needs greater precision, a small Doppler device to check on the baby's heart rate and rhythm.

- **Glucose tolerance test:** A test in which the mother has to fast before her blood is taken and then have blood taken again over the course of several hours while she drinks a sugar solution. This can be boring and annoying for your partner, so try to be there with her. The test checks for gestational diabetes, a condition in which the mother's blood glucose is too high, potentially resulting in the baby having low blood sugar or jaundice.

- **Multiple markers:** Blood tests that screen for hormones and genetic markers that might signal the need for further testing.

- **Nucal translucency screening:** An OB/GYN can combine this special ultrasound test with additional blood screening to look for extra copies of certain chromosomes in the fetus. Called *trisomies,* these extra chromosomes can lead to Down syndrome, congenital heart defects, and other problems.

During pregnancy, your partner will have a vaginal exam with some regularity. Some men get upset or uncomfortable when witnessing their partners' vaginal exams. (She may be quick to claim that having the doctor stick his hand up her innards is far more uncomfortable for her than for you.)

Your reaction isn't surprising, though. After all, you're not used to anyone else examining her genitals. Some men worry that, during a pelvic exam, the doctor might be getting a cheap thrill or threatening to take advantage of your partner. Before you leap up and shout in protest, consider this: the average obstetrician or gynecologist examines dozens of female pelvises a week. Even if the doctor was titillated by pelvic exams during med school (unlikely), the level of repetition quickly erases any arousal from the practice.

It's kind of like this: I dream of owning a Carrera, even though I've never driven one. Now, imagine I got a job working on Porsche's assembly line by some stroke of luck—or managerial incompetence. Before long, my Carrera obsession would probably fade. I might still find them interesting and enjoy driving my own, but I would find something else to fantasize about.

Pregnant Pause

Amniocenteses is much safer than it used to be, but there still is a very slight chance that it can lead to a miscarriage. If you have concerns, discuss with the doctor whether chorionic villus sampling, nucal translucency screening, or other tests can gather the required information with less risk.

You can take comfort in knowing that some other fathers have the same reaction—and that your newborn baby will make *your* gynecological discomfort irrelevant in a hurry.

Daycare Decisions

Most new parents spend a lot of time and effort balancing money, time, and other factors when choosing where, with whom, and how their children will be cared for.

If you have millions of dollars, never have to work again, and both you and your partner can stay home all the time with your new baby, this next bit may be superfluous. Still, super-rich parents also need time away from baby for their own sanity or to nurture their relationship with each other! And someone has to watch the baby while you go out.

What Are My Options?

You have a number of daycare options:

- Both of you stay home to care for the baby.

- You or your partner work outside the home full time while the other person stays home full time.

- A relative (or relatives) cares for your child in their home or yours.

- You and your partner juggle your work and other responsibilities so you each share at-home child-care responsibilities fully.

- You take your child to a daycare center staffed by a team of child development professionals.

- You take your child to a home-based child care, where an adult cares for a small number of kids in her own residence.

- You hire a nanny who comes to (or lives in) your home to care for your child.

Obviously, some arrangements are a lot more expensive than others. Before your baby's born, take time to think about which of the preceding options works best for your time and budget.

Bringing in a Third Party: Daycare Centers and Nannies

If you and your partner decide your baby needs a daycare center, you may wonder how you can judge which provider is good enough for your baby. This is an area where your parenting instincts and common sense can pull you through. Start by visiting any daycare you consider, whether in a facility or a private home.

Spend time observing how the staff treats the kids, and how the kids treat each other. Are the adult-child interactions loving, nurturing, and conducive to learning and development? Are the surroundings safe? Are there quiet spots where children can sleep peacefully and undisturbed? What is the ratio of adult caregivers to children? Very young children (especially babies) need a greater number of adults to provide adequate care. Of course, better staff-child ratios usually translate into higher costs, making this a tough call.

Just as you did with potential doctors, ask questions. Learn where and how the staff obtained their training, ask how long the provider has been in business, get references (and contact them), and find out if the facility or providers are accredited. When you've narrowed your search, return to the "finalists" a second or third time to see if the additional visits reinforce your first impressions.

As with other professionals, reputable daycare providers are used to answering questions and having prospective parents observe their operations. You can find more guidance and resources from The National Association of Child Care Resource and Referral Agencies at naccrra.org.

If you and your partner decide you want a nanny to care for your child, you have something more complicated to do than figuring out a daycare center. Nannies or nanny agencies should be screened vigilantly. You're likely to be the nanny's direct employer, making you responsible for withholding taxes, providing benefits, and meeting other employment requirements. You can find good advice on getting started at babycenter.com/0_how-to-find-a-good-nanny_5933.bc.

The Least You Need to Know

- You have an important role in picking health-care professionals and where your child is born.
- Make your voice heard to advocate for your partner—and yourself—with doctors, nurses, and other staff at medical facilities.
- You have choices about knowing and revealing your baby's gender.
- Start thinking about and researching daycare options now; aim to get your choice made before the baby arrives.

CHAPTER 8

Preparing Your Home

In This Chapter

- Organizing your baby's room
- Picking a bed for your baby
- Choosing diapers, car seats, furniture, and more
- Saving money through hand-me-downs and free and cheap items
- Picking the best toys for your child

You've probably read or heard about the power of a mother's nesting instincts. Well, fathers have nesting instincts, too. Many of us grew up learning how to use tools and do simple (or complex) building projects. Working in partnership with your partner, you can use these skills to demonstrate and relish your personal nesting instinct.

If you've never had a baby before, it's hard to imagine all the things you'll need around the house to keep the baby warm, fed, safe ... and sleeping undisturbed.

You may already be getting unsolicited advice from family and friends about what you need. The first two questions expectant parents hear are often 1) When is your due date?, and 2) Where do you have a baby registry?

It often seems like there are an infinite number of baby products to purchase and preparations to take care of before your baby arrives. Perhaps it's little comfort, but the number of products and projects is actually about 10 or 15 shy of infinite. It can be confusing, but perspective, common sense, and the information in this chapter can steer you in the right direction.

Babies 'r' Lucrative

I don't know how they do it, but every childbirth magazine and infant gadget manufacturer seems to get a catalogue in your mail a week after your partner's positive pregnancy test. Your inbox, search results, and Facebook pages will see a sudden surge in baby gear marketing pitches. Does the NSA inform the world that you're pregnant?

Many of these marketers are out to make a few bucks by encouraging you (or scaring you) into buying their products and services. The following pitch is fictional, but you're likely to see or hear similar hard sells over the next few months and years:

> Don't let your baby's brain be irreversibly stunted! Get the new Bert and Ernie combination stain-proof bib and MP3 player. Call now and we'll include a FREE download of SpongeBob reading the poetry of Emily Dickinson and Dora the Explorer singing the table of elements! Guaranteed to get your child potty trained and into Harvard, Stanford, or the Sorbonne—or your money back!

Because you're a first-time parent, it's easy for these kinds of pitches to play on your insecurity or inexperience. To help you keep your perspective, check out the nonprofit Campaign for a Commercial-Free Childhood (commercialfreechildhood.org). This group of parents, educators, psychologists, and others provide a steady diet of good ideas for dads and moms and gives you insight on the baby gear marketing machine.

Despite all the marketing hype, you and your partner do have quite a few things to hunt, gather, and assemble. Many first-time parents rely on baby showers and other gift-generating channels for the "gathering" phase. First, though, you should do some preliminary "hunting" so your gift-givers have some direction.

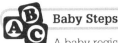 **Baby Steps**

A baby registry is a convenient way for other people to know what you need for your baby. You and your partner first "window shop" in a brick-and-mortar or web store and compile your wish list of specific items by model or SKU number. You then tell friends and families where you've registered. If someone makes a purchase, the store checks that item off your registry list.

Baby gear gathering doesn't need to be a major production. You and your partner get to decide what's essential, keeping in mind that your relationship and the transition to parenthood matters much more than the brand of your stroller.

Organizing the House

How long did it take for you and your partner to work out the "new roommates" kinks once you started living together? That's normal; there's always a period of adjustment with a new roomie, whether in a dorm, apartment, or summer camp cabin.

Well, a newborn is a completely new level of housemate. You can't negotiate, hold a mediation session, or even have a conversation with the baby. Therefore, you have to take charge and make the key decisions about what kind of organization you need in the house before the due date.

It's only a matter of months between the moment you learn you'll be parents and the day you actually become parents. Doctor visits, childbirth classes, baby showers, and buying baby gear will add a lot to your normal schedule. In your excitement, you may take on a large baby prep project—like remodeling a wing of the house—that morphs into a Franken-design Monster.

Based on conversations with hundreds of parents, let me share a few general guidelines for this process:

- **Keep things safe.** This includes you; after all, baby's safety depends on yours. Make sure any items or changes you make aren't potentially harmful to you, your partner, and your baby.

- **Keep things simple.** Your baby won't notice or care about any huge remodeling you did, so don't go overboard with changes.

- **Keep your eye on the ball.** Fixing up your home is less important than preparing yourself and your partner emotionally and psychologically for becoming parents.

- **Keep together.** You and your partner should work as a team to plan and create the baby's room. You'll both have to compromise, and you may carry more of the load when her energy lags. It's just one more way pregnancy mimics parenting!

- **Keep perspective.** Once you can stare into your baby's eyes, her beauty will surpass any scrimshawing or sponge painting you did (or didn't do) in the nursery. And by the time she cares about the wall coverings, it'll be time to redo them anyway.

Don't let dreaming determine your plans for readying your home for a newborn—prioritize how you invest your time and resources. Remember, you need energy left over for labor, delivery, and bringing baby home.

Creating a Nursery

Your first priority is creating a place where the baby can sleep safely and undisturbed. Start by examining your home's layout. Can you transform an entire room of your house into the nursery? Will you have to squeeze the crib into a corner of your apartment? Either option can work, as long as you're realistic about what you need. After you settle on the nursery's location, give the room a good scrubbing and assemble the furniture.

Pregnant Pause

Nursery design usually requires compromise and communication between you and your partner. Do you go for flowery or stick with a spare look? Don't belabor the discussion, but be forewarned: you're asking for trouble if you ignore or dis your partner's nursery desires. Your mutual bottom line is making a dedicated space of peace and quiet that allows the baby to sleep, and gives you a break to do something else—like the dishes!

If you've ever had your kitchen remodeled, you've heard contractors say the best layout requires no more than two steps between the sink, stove, dishwasher, and the counters you use most often. Use the same principle for the nursery, remembering how much you'll have to handle in there when you're tired and juggling in the dark.

Visualize how you will use the nursery space on a daily basis, and consider drawing out a floor plan. You want to be sure you're adapting to the space in ways that maximize your safety and convenience as you move around with the baby. For example, you should have sufficient light on the changing table to see what you're doing but keep the crib in dim light so your baby's sleep isn't disturbed. Also, don't place the changing table in a spot where you're banging your elbow into the wall while you work. And for safety's sake, avoid putting a crib or changing table within reach of a radiator or curtain cords.

When it comes to painting or putting in floor and wall surfaces, make sure whatever you decide on is easy to clean. You'll drop and spill things. The baby will spit up. It'll be much easier to clean up these messes from linoleum than deep-pile carpet. And speaking of floors and paint, flooring adhesives, new carpeting, and paint produce gasses and fumes that can harm pregnant women and newborns. Therefore, leave plenty of time for the fumes to dissipate before your due date, and be proactive (for example, with a window fan) if you have to.

Childproofing

Early on, your infant won't be getting from one place to another unless you carry her. Still, it's a good idea to childproof your entire home *before* you have the baby. There's not much free time afterward, and before you turn around, she'll be exploring electric outlets with her fingers and crawling into cabinets (she'll pick the one where you store the Clorox first).

You can get childproofing materials at most hardware, department, and toy stores. If you like shopping online, Google "child safety kit" and you'll get sites that sell whole packages. As with anything about children, there are tons of products and alternatives out there. Use your head and your knowledge of how your home is set up when making these purchases. Remember, many of these gadgets will be in place for five years or more, so get ones that will last.

The absolute childproofing essentials are the following:

- Working smoke alarms in every bedroom and other strategic locations in your home. They increase the odds of surviving a fire by 50 percent. For advice on placement, see fire.ca.gov/communications/communications_firesafety_smokealarms.php.

- Outlet covers for *every* outlet in your home.

- One or more safety gates. These portable gates keep a baby from crawling, rolling, or falling through a doorway or down the stairs. They're able to be moved around the house and bring great peace of mind.

- Cupboard/cabinet locks. These small, flexible plastic devices go inside or on doors and keep kids from opening them more than an inch or two. (Until you master their use, they may keep you from opening the door, too, but you'll get the hang of it.)

- Drawer latches. They function like cabinet locks and keep little hands from opening them very far.

- Grip tape or stickers for the floor of the bathtub (or sink, if you use it for bathing) to help prevent the baby from sliding around while soaped up.

- A baby thermometer to take her temperature. These are much more high-tech and easier to use than when we were kids.

- "Sponge" tape or other secure padding to cover sharp edges that an infant or crawling baby can bang into. Make sure there are no loose ends or other spots she can start eating.

- A refrigerator magnet with emergency phone numbers and instructions for baby first aid, CPR, and choking.

 Attention, Please

Some elements of home prep will be a chore, but the process should have healthy dollops of fun, too. Enjoy working alongside your partner, and don't resent it if she's too tired to help. After all, even when you're both cleaning and hammering, she's also growing a baby.

There's certainly no harm in getting things on this "maybe-not-so-essential" list. So, if you have any doubts, get everything:

- Bright stickers for glass doors, so neither the baby nor you (when you're distracted) run into them.

- Roll-up devices for window cords.

- Latches to keep appliance doors (such as for the dishwasher and stove) closed.

- Lock covers for the knobs on your stove and range.

- A lock for your DVD, Blu-Ray, or VCR player. (My friend's toddler put the VCR remote into the tape slot—seemed logical to her, but Dad and Mom never could fish it out.)

- Grips to put over door knobs, making them easier for you to turn while carrying an infant.

- A babysitter instruction book, like the Red Cross' "Babysitter Training Handbook." You can also fill in a template checklist from sites like gerber.com/allstages/parenting_advice/babysitter_guide.aspx. Just be sure you've described your way of doing things and your baby's specific needs.

In addition to buying things, you have to make sure you and your partner have good safety practices. Store all chemicals, household cleaners, medications, and other dangerous substances out of the reach of your child. And don't leave tools, tacks, and nails, lying on the floor; in other words, use your head. Arrange things as if your infant was already a toddler, because those days come fast, and your head is clearer now.

Choosing Your Baby's Bed

With any luck, your baby will spend more time in the nursery than you do—because she'll be asleep in there. Therefore, you have to make sure she has something to sleep in: a crib, cradle, or co-sleeper.

Whatever you choose, it has to be safe (of course). It also has to be built and positioned in a way that won't disrupt the baby's sleep. Those quiet moments are golden for you and her both after another round of feeding, pooping, playing, and crying.

Cradles

Cradles used to be common for infants in their first few weeks and months, but they spark some controversy nowadays. Critics complain that, in a cradle, the baby is at greater risk of being pressed against the sides while she's sleeping; therefore, a full-sized crib is the best option from the beginning.

However, a cradle that doesn't rock back and forth too far can be safe and work fine. The cradle should also have a sturdy bottom with a wide, stable base.

If you'd like more information about cradle safety, check out the Juvenile Products Manufacturers Association's website at jpma.org. There, you can learn about the JPMA seal, which adorns cradles that meet the required safety standards.

Co-Sleepers

A co-sleeper basinet is a three-sided infant bed that attaches to an adult bed. The co-sleeper's fourth side is mostly open to the bed, making it easy for a parent to reach the infant for feeding or soothing. The co-sleeper also has anchoring devices to make sure it doesn't move away from or fall off the bed. In all other respects, it looks and functions like a miniature crib.

Talk through the pros and cons of having a co-sleeper attached to your bed with your partner and your doctor. Then, if you and your partner decide to purchase one, make sure to test the setup well before the baby comes to make sure it's doable.

 Pregnant Pause

Don't confuse co-sleepers with *co-sleeping*, which is when babies sleep in the same bed with their parents. In many non-Western cultures, co-sleeping is very common. And some North American parents favor co-sleeping because it makes nighttime breastfeeding easier, can help infants fall asleep more readily, and promotes closeness with a parent who has been away from the baby at work most of the day.

However, co-sleeping is a controversial practice. The American Academy of Pediatrics (AAP) recommends that babies sleep in the same room as their parents—but not the same bed, as there's a danger of rolling over onto the baby. Meanwhile, proponents argue that parents are aware of their babies' presence in the bed even in sleep, so that's not an issue.

Cribs

Babies don't start sleeping in a regular bed until they are 18 months or older, when they can keep themselves from rolling or falling off a mattress. Until then, your baby will need a crib (even if you start out with a cradle or co-sleeper).

For the first few months, your baby's sleep is her most time-consuming activity—or inactivity, depending on how you look at it. In theory, she'll sleep well enough that you won't need to keep her under constant visual surveillance. If you're certain the crib is safe, that will be the case. But how do you know if the crib you choose is safe? The following are some guidelines to ensure you have a safe crib:

- Make sure the crib is designed properly.

- Assemble the crib correctly and solidly.

- Learn what should and shouldn't go in and on the crib.

- Place the crib in a safe and easy-to-use spot.

Let me now walk you through each of these points in more detail.

Make sure the crib is designed properly. If you buy a new crib, it should meet the safety standards of the U.S. Consumer Products Safety Commission (cpsc.gov) or Health Canada (hc-sc.gc.ca/cps-spc/index-eng.php). Look for a sticker on the crib verifying this.

The crib's framework should be solid; the mattress holder, headboards, and slats should not be loose or jiggle around. Even if the crib is new, check for rough edges, chipped paint, splinters, loose slats, or any other problems.

Federal statutes in Canada and the United States require that a crib's openings be narrow enough to prevent a baby's limbs or head from getting stuck. Therefore, two slats can be no farther than $2\frac{3}{8}$ inches apart from each other. Check to be sure this is the case, and that none of the slats are broken or missing on the crib you choose.

You should also see whether the crib has the proper mattress frame height you and your partner want. Modern cribs allow you to set the height of the mattress frame. Because you two will be reaching in and out of there a lot, you should find a height that can work for both parents and other folks caring for the baby regularly at home. If your partner is substantially shorter than you, or vice versa, compromise—and perhaps some yoga practice—are in order. Like most child-care problems, you'll find ways to figure it out. In this case, it usually makes sense to set the height for the short parent and let the taller one bend over.

Assemble the crib correctly and solidly. A crib can pose a danger if you assemble it incorrectly. Missing, loose, or broken hardware or broken slats can snag the baby, causing injuries—including strangulation. Therefore, you should follow the manufacturer's instructions closely and in order. Also, watch for these problems:

* Broken or bent pieces

* Missing or broken hardware

* Parts that don't fit together properly

* Bolts or screws that don't tighten up snugly

* Loose wood joints

* Headboards with cut-outs or other openings that might snag a baby's limbs or head

* A mattress frame that doesn't sit secure and motionless when attached to the crib posts

* A mattress that leaves large gaps anywhere along its edges

If you decide to buy a used crib or want to use a sentimental hand-me-down, inspect the crib carefully. The corner posts on some older cribs protrude above the side rails. If the protrusion is more than $\frac{1}{16}$ of an inch, the baby's clothes may catch on it and cause problems, especially when she's older and moving around the crib on her own. If it's feasible, saw off the top of the posts so that nothing sticks out, and sand off your handiwork to prevent splinters. Also, depending on its age, an older crib may have slat openings wider than $2\frac{3}{8}$ inches or have lead paint (which can lead to brain damage in infants and children). These are problems you can't readily fix, so consider disposing of the crib. Should you have any other doubts about its sturdiness or safety, don't use it.

Learn what should and shouldn't go in and on the crib. Assembling the crib is just the beginning; you need gear in and on the crib to keep baby safe and comfortable. You also need to make sure you keep potentially harmful items out of the crib. These measures are taken to prevent injury, suffocation, and Sudden Infant Death Syndrome (SIDS). SIDS is the unexplained and unexplainable death of an otherwise healthy infant under 1 year old. While the cause for SIDS is unknown, research does indicate simple steps that can drastically reduce the risk—and they all relate to sleeping.

Attention, Please

Prevention efforts dramatically dropped the incidence of SIDS in the United States to less than 1 child for every 2,000 live births. Still, it is a leading cause of infant death.

Number one is having a firm mattress in your crib, covered with a properly sized *fitted* sheet. Make sure the mattress is designed specifically for the crib you're using. Gaps of more than an inch between the mattress and the crib sides increase the risk of your baby being caught or suffocating.

The U.S. Centers for Disease Control also recommend keeping toys, loose bedding, and soft objects out of the crib. While you may have trouble sleeping without your favorite pillow, infants have no need for them. Pillows fall in the "soft object" category that should be kept away from the baby, especially her face, to avoid suffocation. Overheating also raises risks of suffocation and SIDS, so keep out heavy blankets.

A more minor safety concern you have to deal with is your baby chewing on the crib. Babies make sense of the world by putting pieces of it in their mouths. Soon, she'll be gnawing on your finger, her toys, the dog's toys, and anything else she can reach—including the crib. To prevent her from learning about splinters with her baby gums, make sure the top of the railings have a snugly fitted teething cap.

The U.S. National Institute of Child Health and Human Development has an excellent (and free) online pamphlet on creating safe sleeping environments for babies: nichd.nih.gov/publications/pubs/documents/bts_safe_environment.pdf.

Place the crib in a safe and easy-to-use spot. Imagine carrying the baby in the dark around the nursery putting her in and taking her out of the crib. Now imagine doing this on little or no sleep while the baby is crying in your arms. Place the crib in an area where cords of any kind are out of the baby's reach—and where adults don't risk tripping over them. And keep the crib on a wall away from radiators, fireplaces, and the like.

Anticipate and remove as many hazards as you can right now, so you don't break something later on. Breaking a piece of furniture is a hassle. Breaking your leg is exponentially more of a hassle when you're trying to care for an infant.

Rocking Chairs or Gliders

Rocking movements help your baby with feeding, soothing, playing, and going to sleep; it mimics her time inside the womb, signaling comfort and safety. That's one reason why so many new parents rely on a rocking chair or glider. The other reason? Rocking calms and comforts your partner and you, too. These two reasons are connected, because your baby is swift to pick up on your tension or anxiety and become tense and anxious herself in response. So if you and your partner are calm, she's calm.

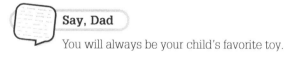

Say, Dad

You will always be your child's favorite toy.

—Vicki Lansky, parenting author

Your choice in rocking chair will depend on your budget and the size of your nursery. You can get a large, upholstered, and "real" piece of furniture that you can use for years, or you can opt for a simpler, less expensive chair. Plain wooden rockers work fine, as long as the construction is solid and the rockers themselves have a short rocking range. Use cushioning and pillows to make sitting more comfortable and to help prop up the baby for feeding.

A glider uses sprigs and hinges underneath the seat to generate a rocking motion. Gliders tend to be more stable than a wooden rocking chair, because they have a rectangular, solid base on the floor that makes the chair more stable. Like a rocking chair, you'll want to make sure you have cushioning for comfort. You'll also want to maintain and clean the gliding mechanism; if it starts squeaking, you may drive yourself and the baby to distraction.

Bath Goodies

Infants get messy when they eat, burp, pee, and poop. The older they get, the more opportunities there are for messes. Therefore, babies need regular baths—in a place that won't endanger her or you. An inexpensive "infant tub" is a small tub you use for babies when they're small; it can be placed in a large sink, countertop, or bathtub.

An infant's skin is very sensitive, so buy mild soaps along with very soft towels and washcloths. Because your baby won't be climbing trees or rolling around in the dirt, you won't have to scrub her clean.

 Pregnant Pause

Safety is a big issue with infant tubs. Keep the tub level on a secure, flat surface, and never leave the baby during a bath. In addition, make sure she is secure within the tub; that may take two sets of hands when she's tiny.

The temperature of baby's bathwater matters a lot, which has led baby superstores to offer a $25 rubber ducky bathwater thermometer. Of course, it's cheaper and more fun to learn how to test the water from a bath-battle-hardened parent (including your own) and buy multiple low-tech rubber duckies for the baby. It's your choice.

When picking a space for the bath and any bath equipment, survey the space to make sure your baby won't be able to reach the faucet, spout, small appliances, or other potential dangers.

The Diaper-Driven Life

Over the next couple of years, your days will be filled with the sweet smells of pee and poop. You'll quickly learn the new parent's mantra: "Diapers: don't leave home without 'em!"

You also need a place to put them and change them on your baby, which is where diaper bags and changing tables come in.

Cloth or Plastic?

A rare parent attempts to raise his infant without diapers. Who wants to carry the baby 24/7, at considerable arms' length, over an easy-to-clean surface? No thanks. Let's look at the different options you have when it comes to what diapers your baby will wear.

Fully disposable diapers are very convenient in the short term. Throw out the dirty diaper and replace it with a new one—no pins, pants, or problems!

Unfortunately, the planet has problems with disposables. They amount to a disproportionate part of the materials entering U.S. landfills—upward of 2 percent of all solid waste. Much of a disposable diaper (at least 30 percent) is made of plastic. And because at least 30 percent of a disposable diaper is made from plastic, which doesn't disintegrate, this waste lasts for centuries in the dump.

Aside from environmental objections, some parents complain that the plastic in disposable diapers chafes their infant's skin and make them sweat. This contributes to diaper rash, particularly when the weather is warm.

"Regular" cloth diapers last a very long time; your kid can even take some to college as dust rags in 18 years. Nowadays, cloth diapers don't require safety pins; instead, a plastic outer cover with Velcro or plastic snaps holds the diaper in place. This ends up making the diaper look like a pair of very short, stuffed shorts.

You can often reuse the cover a few times before washing, especially if there's no poop. If there is poop, cloth diapers take more work than disposables. You have to rinse off the bulk of poop in a toilet, especially after the baby is taking solid food and generating more output.

During your baby's early weeks, you may also need a "snappi"—a simple plastic "gripper" that helps fasten the diaper in place around her little legs before you put on the cover. Or, if you like, you can use safety pins. (Ask your mother for the cute ducky ones you had when you were an infant!)

Cloth diapers are handy for many other purposes, such as burping and wiping up almost anything a baby produces. Cloth also tends to reduce the amount of skin irritation and diaper rash, especially if you use the unbleached variety made from organic cotton. These are a bit more expensive but very sturdy.

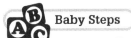

Baby Steps

If you can afford it or can get it as the ideal baby gift, a diaper service can whisk away the dirty cloth diapers and replace them with clean ones.

Cloth diapers don't generally add to the solid waste stream. Even if they enter a landfill, cloth diapers will eventually degrade. But they do have an environmental impact. You use water and detergent to wash diapers, and manufacturers use resources to make and distribute them. Plus, some argue that disposable and cloth diapers use roughly the same amount of resources to make. Even if that's true, the long-term disposal impact is greater for plastic diapers than cotton.

Hybrid diapers combine a disposable inner liner with cloth outer "shorts" that hold everything together. The liner peels off and, because it's made of biodegradable fibers, you can dispose of it safely. Fasteners (such as Velcro) keep the cover in place and add to convenience.

The hybrid is almost as easy to use as a fully disposable diaper but with much less trash. You can reuse the covers several times before they need washing. However, hybrids are more expensive than cloth diapers or disposables.

Pocket diapers have a waterproof cover sewn to an inside polyester fleece pocket. You stuff a microfiber absorbing layer into the fleece "pocket" before use and then remove it before washing. The fleece helps wick moisture away from your baby's skin.

One nice thing about pocket diapers is you can stuff a bunch of them in the morning and have a ready-to-wear supply for your baby all day. The biggest disadvantage? You have to wash them after a single use, and the synthetic fabrics in pocket diapers can be harder to clean.

All-in-twos are another type of pocket diaper. This style uses a cloth insert, which you can remove and wash separately. That means you can (usually) use the rest of the cover more than once before washing.

All-in-ones are cloth diapers with a waterproof cover and absorbent liner sewn together in one piece. They are convenient to use and allow you to wash everything together. However, because the absorbent layer is sandwiched up against the waterproof cover, some brands can be hard to dry. Look for a variety where the layers can open up when you put them in the dryer.

Changing Tables

Changing tables are a popular item on baby registries. Retailers carry changing tables of various sizes, storage spaces, accoutrements, and prices.

A store-bought changing table has a belt that gently straps the baby down so she can't roll off the table. It also has a waterproof pad (for comfort) and a low barrier around the changing surface (for added safety).

 Pregnant Pause

While the safety strap won't allow your baby to fall off the table, it won't stop her from moving around. Therefore, you should always have a hand on her to keep her still.

You can also convert a table or dresser that you already own into a changing table, as long as it is solidly built and has a flat working surface. If you decide to adapt your own furniture, make sure it has similar safety features to a store-bought model. Ideally, it should have room for plenty of diapering supplies on, under, or nearby it.

You also want to make sure a trashcan and (if you're using cloth diapers) a diaper pail are within easy reach.

In a perfect world, the changing table can sit at an ideal height for you and your partner at the same time. In the real world, though, height is seldom a key factor in choosing a mate. Therefore, just like with crib height, you may have to adjust.

Diaper Bags

Smart parents enjoy leaving their own house sometimes, and they often bring the baby with them! While it's terribly inconvenient, your baby doesn't hold off being hungry or defer defecating when you walk out the front door. That's why you need a diaper bag.

Because it will hold more than diapers, a diaper bag has to be roomy and easy to carry. As with the changing table, you can adapt a bag you already own or purchase one designed specifically for this purpose.

Following is a list of essentials that will go in your diaper bag. When looking for the right bag, make sure it can hold all of these items:

- More than one disposable diaper
- More than one cloth diaper, towel, or soft rag for burping and cleanup
- Travel-size containers of baby wipes and ointment
- A waterproof pad or blanket to use for changing diapers on any flat surface
- One or more bottles of formula or breast milk (if your partner and her breasts aren't along for the ride)
- At least two pacifiers
- A few small toys to entertain and distract the baby

It's also wise to have a simple way to carry dirty diapers home with you, so see if the bag you're looking at has a place to store them. Most modern diaper bags have a waterproof compartment.

Car Safety Seats

Virtually all parents must transport their babies in a vehicle at some point or another. Therefore, before your baby arrives, you need to have a car seat and know how to use it.

Car seats form a protective barrier that absorbs the force of a crash and prevents your baby from flying around or out of the vehicle. While using a car safety seat doesn't guarantee your baby will never suffer any harm in an accident, it dramatically reduces the risk.

Why Use One?

Driving an infant without a car seat is illegal everywhere in Canada and the United States. In fact, no hospital will let you drive a newborn home unless she's in a car seat. This change in public policy has rapidly reduced—but not eliminated—the number of children killed in traffic accidents.

The issue here, however, is not keeping you from getting a ticket, being hassled by a discharge nurse, or learning some new statistics— it's to keep your baby from harm.

Nothing can substitute for a car seat. No matter how strong you are, your strength alone can't protect your child through holding or restraining her during an accident, even at relatively slow speeds.

There are no reasons or excuses for failing to put your child in a functioning, correctly installed child safety seat every single time that child is in a vehicle. None.

Car Seat Options and Costs

Like other baby stuff, a car seat can be a substantial investment. You have several choices when purchasing a new car safety seat. The cost differences are almost all related to how convenient the seat is for parents.

The so-called combo seat is more expensive than a simple infant seat. It pops out of a base secured to the vehicle's back seat. The benefit of this is being able to move the baby without having to get her out of the seat itself. Of course, you still have to strap and unstrap her, but that's easier to do in the house, rather than when bending over into the middle of the car's backseat.

Once you remove the combo seat, you can then use it as an infant seat in the house or snap it into a companion stroller and wheel it away. These strollers come in many models and with many options (more on strollers later in this chapter).

A "convertible" car seat (which may also have "combo" features) has additional settings that can be adjusted when your child is large enough to move to a front-facing position; thus, you don't have to buy another car seat as the child grows. In addition, it typically has higher height and weight limits for the rear-facing position, allowing you to keep your child rear-facing for a longer period of time.

The least expensive option is an infant-only car seat, which only faces backward—and doesn't attach to a stroller or have any other "combo" uses.

 Pregnant Pause

Safety experts recommend using a rear-facing seat while your child weighs less than 20 pounds. After that, she'll need to be in a front-facing car seat up to 40 pounds and then a safety booster seat beyond that.

If you buy a new car seat, be sure to fill in and return the enclosed registration form, so you'll get word of any future warnings or recalls on your model.

You can spend hundreds of dollars on a high-end combination car seat/stroller, and hundreds more on accessories for it. The costs can add up quickly. For example, can you put the car seat in a plastic garbage bag (rather than a $70 travel bag) on those days you need to carry it through the rain? Can you use a less-expensive car seat and stroller, even if it means transferring the baby back and forth between them (while getting to hold and chatter with him each time)? When buying new, think it through before making your choice.

Buying secondhand or borrowing could work, but it requires you to do some detective work. When thinking of buying or borrowing a car seat, make sure the following is true:

* The car seat hasn't been in an accident, even a little one.

* The car seat has no damage, no matter how small.

* The car seat isn't too old.

Car seats have expiration dates, usually five or six years from the date of manufacture. If the seat is older than this, it may not meet current safety standards or have lost some of its structural reliability. And Saint Louis Children's Hospital's Sharon Rau warns there's no sure way to trace the history of a used car seat: "A crash or fender bender can damage the integrity of the seat even if you can't see it from the outside."

Fortunately, many hospitals and law enforcement agencies offer programs where you can rent a child safety seat for the first few years of your child's life. Some car and health insurance companies have occasional free or discounted car seat offers, too. Call yours and ask.

If you have questions about whether your used or new seat is up to par, call the National Highway Traffic Association's Vehicle Safety Hotline at 1-800-424-9393 (1-800-424-9153 for people with hearing impairments). There's no room for shortcuts on this one. Your child's life is worth having a good car seat.

Proper Use

The day you leave the hospital, and for many months thereafter, you'll put the baby in a rear-facing car seat. This provides the most protection for smaller children in an accident.

It's also critical to secure the car seat in the rear of the car, ideally in the middle of the backseat. Why not the front seat? Car companies made airbags standard equipment more than 15 years ago. Airbags save many adult lives, but they are deadly for infants and children. In the nanoseconds after a collision, the passenger-side airbag blows out of the dashboard at 200 miles an hour. That force can kill a child in the front seat, no matter which way the car seat is facing.

While the proper car seat setup means your baby can't see you if you're driving, that won't kill her. Riding in front where you can see her might. So before your baby's born, learn the proper methods for securing your baby in her car seat.

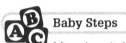
Baby Steps

Many hospitals, local fire departments, and AAA offices can instruct you on how to install, use, and remove your car seat safely. You can also find additional car seat inspection sites at nhtsa.gov/cps/cpsfitting/index.cfm.

For Saner Sailing

To keep the baby happy—and to keep you from losing it—consider investing in a stroller, play yard, swaddle, and other smaller items that make carting around your baby a little easier.

Strollers

Whether you're strolling or running, wheeling the baby around town is fun and stimulating for you, your partner, and your infant. When sitting in the stroller, your baby sees new sights and takes in the world. Meanwhile, neighbors and perfect strangers will stop and strike up conversations as they ooh and aah over your cutie pie.

Once again, retailers offer you a range of functionality, style, weight, and cost in strollers. As I mentioned earlier, "combo" strollers have frames large enough to carry the car seat. So-called "jogging" strollers have sturdy frames and only three wheels, so you can steer more easily while bringing the baby along for your exercise runs. And "umbrella" strollers (so-named because they fold up somewhat like a bumbershoot) have a smaller frame and wheelbase, making them easier to maneuver in small spaces.

Several factors are likely to influence your decision about which stroller to purchase or borrow—and whether you might need more than one:

- Does the stroller adjust for adults of different heights?

- Does it have other features (for example, storage pouches, pockets, and cup holders) you feel you need?

- Will it collapse and fit easily in the trunk or back of your car?

- Is it too heavy for a smaller adult (for example, your partner, you, or a grandparent) to fold up and carry?

- Is it sturdy enough to handle the environments of your daily routine (for example, sidewalks, jogging routes, and hiking trails)?

- Will it maneuver into and around your home in the way you want?

- How will it affect the amount of effort you put into transferring the baby to and from the car seat, home, and other places?

- If you use public transit, can you get it on and off the bus or train easily?

- Does it meet current safety standards?

Start with some research shopping—trying different strollers without making a purchase immediately. Wheel a stroller into a crowded space that replicates the grocery store or coffee shop you visit regularly. You'll be using the stroller a lot, so find one that is comfortable for you, doesn't have extra stuff (and weight) you don't need, and is easy to steer and store.

You can also ask your friends and family what type of strollers worked best for their lifestyles and situations. You can then compare models and read user reviews online.

Practice using your new stroller before you buy, so you know you're operating it correctly. To make sure you know all the safety steps involved in operating a stroller, check out JPMA's "Safety House" website: jpma.org/content/parents/safety-house.

Swaddles

A baby can have involuntary, reflexive muscle movements that make her appear to be startled (which, sometimes, she is). When she startles in her sleep, she'll often wake up before she's fully rested. Swaddling cuts down on the side effects of infant startles. The swaddle holds the baby's limbs close to her body, minimizing movement, keeping her warm, and helping to simulate her womb experience.

You can buy a variety of swaddles, which are basically a combination sack/blanket specifically designed to wrap the baby easily. Swaddles use Velcro tabs and come in sizes to fit a growing baby. You can also use a so-called "receiving blanket" to swaddle your infant, although that takes a little more work.

 Baby Steps

To learn how to swaddle your baby, watch an instructive swaddling slideshow at mayoclinic.com/health/how-to-swaddle-a-baby/MY01766. Or see 5-day-old Naya and her dad demonstrate swaddling with a simple baby blanket at youtu.be/W4SnaQ1DVJM.

The American Academy of Pediatrics recommends swaddling only for the first two months. This is due to concerns about (and debate over) swaddling as a risk for SIDS once an infant can roll over on her own.

Carriers

Manufacturers offer you a wide variety of products that perform the function of a papoose—the traditional child carrier named after the Narragansett word for "child."

Modern carriers allow you to carry your baby on your back or your front, with the baby facing inward or outward. She'll get lots of stimulation and draw lots of attention when facing out. When facing in, you and she will get lots of face time and snuggling action. Both ways will be good for baby and you!

Still other models are dual purpose. You can configure them to wear on your front or your back. As with other baby gear, the easier-to-use (and adjust) carriers are generally more expensive.

Another type of carrier uses a long piece of fabric that you fold around your shoulders, torso, and waist to hold the baby. Commonly known as Mobys (after the popular Moby Wrap), there's a learning curve for you.

Sort of like learning to ride a bike, you'll practice several times (and feel like an idiot) until you get the hang of it. Eventually, the baby will have a warm, secure place to snuggle, your hands will be free, and (if you did it correctly) your back won't hurt.

Wait until the baby can hold her head up for a good amount of time before purchasing or using a model with the pouch in the back, as the back pouches tend to be more heavy duty. Some of them are even designed for hikes and camping. (Camping with diapers is the definition of extreme camping, but some people do it.)

Portable Play Yards

The baby's crib is too large and unwieldy to be portable. So what do you do when journeying to Grandpa and Grandma's house? A play yard is a good solution. Play yards (what my parents called *playpens*) are relatively lightweight and collapse for easy transportation.

A play yard functions like a small crib. Your infant will be able to sleep comfortably on its mattress, as long as the mattress fits snugly (just as your crib mattress should). Instead of slats, a play yard has mesh on its sides. Make sure the mesh holes aren't more than

¼ inch in diameter; otherwise, they could trap your baby's fingers or limbs.

As your baby grows and begins to sit up, the play yard will also function as a safe, contained place for her to, well, play! It will even hold (and entertain) a baby who's crawling and learning to stand up, although usually for only short periods.

When shopping for a play yard, ask similar questions as you would when looking for a stroller. Can you, your partner, and other adults assemble, disassemble, and carry the play yard? Does it fit in the car? Will it hold up under the additional movement and stress of a standing, active baby?

Safe operation is once again key. After you bring it home and set it up, you shouldn't use string or rope to hang toys or anything else to the side of the play yard or across the top. In addition, check the mesh and railings for any holes or tears (and if you find any, fix them!).

Before you use a play yard for the first time, open and collapse it a few times. It may take a few tries to get the hang of making everything secure when it's up and getting everything where it belongs when knocking down. Take it from me: I bought a play yard to have at our house for my grandson. The way it unfolded and folded looked extraordinarily obvious to me, but after 30 minutes of sweat and frustration, I had to read the directions.

Hand-Me-Downs, Freebies, and Cheapies

Buying all this baby gear gets expensive in a hurry. Don't be timid about asking friends and relatives for hand-me-downs. You can also tap into Craigslist, Freecycle, thrift stores, and garage sales. But use common sense and keep baby's safety first.

For example, St. Louis Children's Hospital safety expert Sharon Rau recommends you avoid putting your infant in a previously used car seat or crib. Safety standards continue to be updated on those items, and you can't be sure that older models fit the bill. Similarly, a used crib mattress may not fit snugly into the crib you have, which can be dangerous for a sleeping baby.

 Baby Steps

You can listen to Rau discuss secondhand baby gear at youtu.be/aZyF8jm15JY. You can also find other useful info on baby health and safety from Rau and her colleagues at stlouischildrens.org/health-resources/healthinfo/wellness-development.

You should also check for stability and safety in used high chairs, strollers, Bumbo seats, and so on. Previously worn clothes are fine, as long as they you clean them thoroughly; however, avoid any infant clothes with drawstrings hanging from them.

When thinking about baby gear, remember this wise old saying: "your child needs your presence more than he needs your presents." Nothing you buy can replace your healthy involvement in your child's life.

Buying the Right Toys

From the get-go, you will need to put thought into what toys you choose for—and keep away from—your child.

Over the course of her childhood, the average U.S. child spends far more time in front of screens (TVs, tablets, smartphones, computers, and so on) than she does in school or interacting with her family. That is a radical shift in how a child "plays" compared to 25, 50, or 100,000 years ago.

By most measures, this shift has been decidedly unhealthy for the physical, intellectual, psychological, emotional, and social development of children. Skyrocketing rates of childhood obesity and attention-deficit/hyperactivity disorder (ADHD) are only the beginning.

Most electronic toys and entertainment provide external stimulation with narrow (if any) ways for the child to use them, which research shows tends to dull the child's senses and imagination, encourages passivity, and eats up time that could be spent interacting with others. The American Academy of Pediatrics also strongly recommends no screen time of any kind until a child is at least 2 years old. (See aap.org/en-us/advocacy-and-policy/aap-health-initiatives/Pages/Media-and-Children.aspx for more information.)

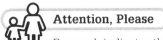

Attention, Please

Research indicates that children play less creatively with toys based on media characters.

Plus, you've probably heard many veteran parents tell the tale of staying up late to assemble some high-tech toy, only to have the child ignore it for hours of play with the empty box the toy came in. Nature communicates an important lesson in that amusing story.

So how do you avoid these issues? This is actually very simple and practical to accomplish. During your child's first few years, limit the number of electronic toys and objects in her life. (Squeaky squeeze animal, yes; iPad, no.) Even though electronic media and toys are here to stay, you can work actively to provide your child with an "unplugged" space, where her development is stimulated naturally, away from the bombardment of hyperkinetic electronic media and toys.

Appropriate toys for your baby's first few months are simple and straightforward. You'll need (and might easily get as gifts) rattles, rings, and other things she can suck on. You can also hang (where the baby can see and not touch) bright pictures of faces and patterns. Brightly colored vinyl and cardboard infant books are fun to play with and help set a reading pattern now and later. (Yes, you should start reading to your infant even before she has any idea what you're doing.)

Once your child is older, she'll have enough imagination to make anything and anyone out of blocks, dolls, and stuffed animals—and make anything happen with them. So mix in books, music, physical activity, and human interaction, and you have a child whose brain and social skills are continually stimulated from without and within.

Setting aside the heavily marketed array of electric toys may seem like a radical step. Perhaps, by some standards, it is. However, by the standard of your child's well-being and future, it's the smart step to take.

The Least You Need to Know

- Prepare the house as much as you can before the baby comes and consumes all of your energy and attention.
- Common sense, advice from veteran parents, and online resources can help you shop smartly for the equipment you and your baby need.
- Hand-me-down and used baby gear is fine, as long as it's safe and in good shape.
- Buy toys that will stimulate your child's imagination and don't require a lot of batteries or assembly.

Preparing Your Legal, Financial, and Work Life

In This Chapter

- Taking care of legal issues before the baby arrives
- Planning your parental finance approach
- Finding a family-work balance

If you need a break from reading about the emotional and psychological aspects of becoming a dad, this chapter may be just right for you.

Planning budgets, insurance coverage, and work schedules isn't very sexy or dramatic. Nevertheless, you have to take on these tasks in order to prepare for family life. It's easy to ignore or delay all this in the excitement and flurry of the pregnancy. However, just remember that you'll have considerably less time to handle this *after* your baby is born.

In this chapter, I go through the legal, financial, and work preparations you have to make before your baby is born.

Legal Issues

Once your baby is born, his legal status changes. He becomes a person under the law, with certain rights and (already) certain responsibilities. For example, the law says he needs a birth certificate.

The legal status, rights, and obligations of you and your parenting partner change, too. Because you're both adults, those rights and responsibilities are more complicated than for your baby.

Pregnant Pause

This chapter discusses complex issues with major consequences for your life, but it doesn't cover them in minute detail. If you have questions or need further information, contact an attorney, financial advisor, or other specialist.

Taxes and Government

As a student of history, I know that fear of government has ebbed and flowed many times over the years. Some folks are leery of the government and believe it is unwise (or even dangerous) to have a Social Security number or other government-issued identification. However, in my humble opinion, history also shows that—as far as inherently imperfect human endeavors go—the United States and Canada are model systems of government for responding to their citizens and maintaining peace. Your child is considerably more vulnerable if you try to hide his existence from the government, because it complicates his access to important rights and services, including the right to be a full member of his local and national community. Plus, without this information, you won't be able to claim the income tax benefits that come with having a child.

If your child is a U.S. citizen, you'll need to get him a Social Security number shortly after he's born. When getting information for the birth certificate, the hospital will usually ask if you want to apply for the baby's Social Security number. (If they don't ask, tell them you want to do it anyway.) On the application, you'll have to provide the Social Security numbers for you and your partner. The state agency that issues birth certificates will share your child's information with the Internal Revenue Service. The government will then assign your baby a number and mail his Social Security card directly to you.

In the United States, you'll be able to claim a "personal exemption" for your child, provided you aren't already subject to the Alternative Minimum Tax. The exemption value usually increases slightly each year (for example, the $3,900 deduction for 2013 was $100 higher than the one in 2012). To do this, you'll simply subtract the exemption amount from your adjusted gross income, in effect reducing your taxable income.

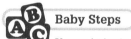 **Baby Steps**

If your baby is born at 11:55 P.M. on December 31, you'll still be able to claim his exemption on your U.S. tax return for that year. If he's born six minutes later, though, you won't be able to claim him until you file your return for the new year.

If you and your partner aren't legally married, even if you live together all year, only one of you will be able to deduct for the baby. According to the IRS, to qualify for the exemption, your child must live with you more than half of the year. You can learn more about U.S. tax credits and deductions for children at irs.gov/Credits-&-Deductions.

In Canada, your baby needs only a provincial birth certificate; she won't get her federal social insurance number until she grows up and gets her first job. Canadian law lets one parent claim a child as a dependent, although the dollar amount is less than in the United States. As a Canadian, you can claim additional tax deductions, such as for being a single parent or for certain child-care expenses. Federal and provincial governments also offer direct, tax-free payments to eligible families to help with the cost of raising children. You can learn more about Canadian tax credits and deductions for children at cra-arc.gc.ca/ndvdls-fmls/menu-eng.html.

Married or Not, Here I Come

If you're married and listed as "father" on your baby's birth certificate, the law presumes you're the biological father. However, things are not so straightforward if you and your partner aren't married.

In the United States, state and federal governments award privileges to married people while withholding the same benefits from the unmarried (including the tax breaks I just discussed). While the number of parents who aren't married continues to grow, the law continues to operate with the supposition that children are (and ought to be) born in a family formed by legal marriage between the parents. This is because marriage is a legal contract, which makes things clearer in the eyes of the law. It simplifies issues with employers, insurance companies, the IRS, hospitals, schools, social service agencies, and a host of other people and institutions you'll encounter over the years.

In Canada, fathers who live with—and provide support for—their child (whether married to the mother or not) can claim federal benefits for the child and take paid parental leave of up to 35 weeks. If he is the primary caregiver, a Canadian dad may be eligible for additional government services.

 Pregnant Pause

If you use a surrogate for any part of conception, make sure you're dealing with a reputable agency, so there are no doubts about your role as the legal parent. You also want to address all the current and future issues that may arise, such as genetic disorders or a child's desire to contact his surrogate mother or sperm donor when he's older. Consult an attorney experienced in these issues to help assure that the law will treat you like a biological parent in all areas, even divorce and custody.

If you and your partner aren't married, you need to check right away to see whether your health insurance carrier will cover the expenses related to the birth. Some insurance companies do, while others don't; the same holds true for publicly subsidized health insurance. It depends on how the insurer defines terms like *household*, *family*, and *spouse*; you don't automatically get the same presumption of rights for your family as a married couple. That may not be fair, but it is reality. You should also alter your will and any life insurance policies to list your child as a beneficiary (more on this later in the chapter).

If you're an unmarried dad, you'll have to establish paternity to prove that you're the legal father of your child. If you aren't married to your partner, the law in many states assumes your child doesn't have a legal father. This means, unless you and your partner take explicit steps to establish paternity, your name won't appear on your child's birth certificate, which can affect your legal rights to custody. Plus, because widely held social attitudes continue to see women as primarily (if not completely) responsible for raising children, laws, policies, and customs reflect those attitudes, sanctifying a biological mother's ability to manage her child's life. By establishing your paternity, you'll make sure the law recognizes your rights as a parent and show you want to be a part of your child's life. This principle holds true under both Canadian and U.S. law.

For example, if your relationship with your partner breaks up before or after your baby's birth, you'll need established paternity to assert your rights and responsibilities fully regarding child support, visitation, custody, and other issues concerning your child.

The first step to establishing paternity will be getting your name on the baby's birth certificate. You'll be able to do this when filling out the forms in the hospital. There's some urgency when it comes to getting this done, because if you wait, you'll have to amend the birth certificate—meaning extra forms, extra time, filing fees, and more. Waiting creates unnecessary hassle and will leave you legally vulnerable, so don't do it.

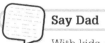 **Say Dad**

With kids, the days are long, but the years are short.

—John Leguizamo, actor

Unfortunately, your name on the birth certificate won't necessarily provide enough legal protection for your father-child bond in every state or province. Therefore, you may need to take additional steps to establish paternity sooner rather than later (you can do it later, but that makes it unnecessarily complicated).

Most states participate in the Paternity Opportunity Program (POP) or an equivalent. POPs use a standard "Certificate of Parentage" form to make it easier for parents to acknowledge paternity voluntarily. (Some states and jurisdictions call this a *paternity declaration form*.) You can usually find the form at the following places:

- The hospital where your child was born

- Local registrars of births and deaths (usually found in your city hall or county government headquarters)

- Local or county child support, child welfare, or family services departments

- Local courts (which may be known as county, parish, district, circuit, or superior courts, depending on where you live)

By signing and submitting an official paternity declaration form, you'll help your child gain the same rights and privileges of a child born within a marriage, including the following:

- Access to important family medical records

- Medical benefits from a live-away (or noncustodial) parent

- Financial support from both parents

- The emotional and psychological benefit of knowing who both of his parents are

There may be times when a paternity declaration form and your name on the birth certificate still won't be enough for a particular institution or a legal situation. In those cases, you'll need to take the additional step of having a paternity test. This one-time test will require a DNA sample from you and the newborn (usually a swab taken from inside the cheek) for analysis by a laboratory. The paternity test will provide documentation that your child shares your DNA, which will prove your paternity in a court of law.

You can have a paternity test done locally or use labs you find on the internet. When taking a paternity test, only use a laboratory accredited by the American Association of Blood Banks. You can locate a nearby facility for genetic testing at their website: aabb.org.

Issues for Same-Sex Partners

In the United States, gay fathers don't have the same legal protections as nongay fathers, in large part because they cannot marry each other in most states. U.S. Supreme Court decisions in 2013 effectively legalized gay marriage in California (the most-populous state) and overturned key provisions of the federal Defense of Marriage Act (DOMA). So far, the DOMA changes appear to bring the most immediate benefits to federal employees, including members of the military. This development does nothing, however, for gay dads planning to have children, if they work outside the federal government or live in the majority of states that still restrict family rights for same-sex parents.

In Canada, gay marriage is legal; homosexual men and women can marry their partners and obtain all the rights (including the right to divorce) as married heterosexual couples. However, the rights of unmarried gay parents are less consistent. For example, gay parents who live together have the same rights and responsibilities as heterosexual common law partners under British Columbia and Ontario provincial statute but may not in other provinces that haven't passed similar laws; therefore, some rights may have to be obtained in a courtroom.

A gay dad can have a hard time getting health insurance and other employment-related benefits for his child if the child isn't his biologically. Even when a same-sex couple adopts, some states recognize only one of the adults as the adoptive parent, leaving the other parent without legal standing. In other states, both men can petition for a joint adoption. If one of you is the biological donor to this pregnancy, the nonbiological dad may be able to legally adopt the child—but this depends on the laws in your state.

Under the law, the "legally recognized" dad is the only one allowed to decide on the health, education, and well-being of the couple's children. If the legally recognized father dies or is incapacitated, his partner may not have the right to become the legal guardian for their child.

Without the legal presumption that both fathers are legal parents, it's crucial to have written agreements about what you want for your child. Obviously, you need a clearly articulated will for the worst situations, but you also need documents that deal with everyday situations (for example, giving your partner "permission" to make medical decisions for the baby if you aren't there in the emergency room).

 Say, Dad

I am 30 years old, and I still find great power in my own dad telling me it's possible; I can do it.

—Dan Pearce, fathering author

Draw up a parenting agreement explicitly stating that both of you accept and welcome the responsibilities of raising this child, agree to share the rights of parents, and commit to maintaining your co-parenting duties even if your personal relationship changes or ends. The website nolo.com/legal-encyclopedia/parenting-agreements-29565.html has an agreement geared for a couple in the process of breaking up, but you could use the same form to clarify things earlier in your parenting relationship.

You and your partner should also update or create your wills (more on this later in the chapter) so the court knows who you choose to be your child's guardian should one or both of you die.

For more information about legal steps you and your partner can take as parents, a good resource is Lambda Legal (lambdalegal.org), a national nonprofit that uses litigation, education, and public policy to gain legal and civil rights for lesbians, gay men, bisexuals, the transgendered, and people with HIV or AIDS.

Financial Issues

Most parents who start a family are young and not exactly rich. Your income and living expenses have a big impact on life with a baby. No matter what your financial status, you can make plans to meet your new family's needs, set priorities for the future, and anticipate common life events.

Family Budgeting

I don't like having limitations on how much I can buy ... or on how much employers pay me. How about you? It's human nature to "want it all," as if we never entirely get past being a terrible 2-year-old. Ironically, this human trait is an excellent reason to have a family budget. For example, a budget can help you manage the temptation to buy every baby gadget that comes down the pike or to keep spending hundreds of dollars on video games each month.

Budgeting helps you recognize the more pressing priorities your new baby brings when it comes to "investing" your money. There will be one-time expenses like a crib and car seat (see Chapter 8) you have to meet even before your baby comes. Afterward, there are ongoing expenses, such as clothing (babies dirty up and then grow out of their clothes with alarming rapidity) and child care.

 Say, Dad

Mother Nature, in her infinite wisdom, has instilled within each of us a powerful biological instinct to reproduce; this is her way of assuring that the human race, come what may, will never have any disposable income.

—Dave Barry, author

So before your baby arrives, sit down with your partner and create a budget. List your take-home pay (after taxes) and an honest, realistic list of your expenses. Then add in your estimate of the new expenses (one-time and ongoing) associated with having a child.

This is not an easy process, because it almost always involves deciding to "cut" something—say, eating out as often as you're used to doing. The budget helps you assess the difference between your "needs" and your "I wants." Budgeting can also reveal incentives and simple methods to save money by buying secondhand, clipping coupons, using shopping lists (they reduce "impulse" purchases), and comparison shopping.

The financial decisions you make (and the way you make them) say a lot about your values and what's important to you. So treat budgeting as a learning experience. You can find family budgeting tips and templates online at parentsconnect.com/parents/family-finance/family-budget/how-to-create-budget.html and kidmoney.about.com/od/newbaby/ht/budgetnewbaby.htm.

By getting a draft budget down on paper, you'll avoid flying blind financially and be able to prioritize things so the baby will get what he needs when he arrives and in the future.

If you still need financial help making ends meet for your growing family, check out the federal WIC (which stands for the unfortunately gendered title "Women, Infants, and Children") program at fns.usda.gov/wic/. The WIC program helps lower-income families during pregnancy and until the child is 5 years old by supplementing them with nutritious foods (including formula, if needed) and providing nutrition counseling and referrals to other support services.

For a summary of Canada's federal assistance for low-income families, visit servicecanada.gc.ca/eng/audiences/families/benefits.shtml.

Insurance Coverage for Your Family

If you haven't done so already, line up health insurance as early as possible for you and your partner. You can start by checking with your employer to see what kind of insurance they offer (if any) and how you can sign up. Make sure your child can be covered in your policy, too, since there will be plenty of doctor's visits ahead. Even if he ends up being insanely healthy, he'll need check-ups, vaccinations, and the like, and they all cost money.

If you have family coverage, make sure to notify your health insurance company soon after the baby is born. That will get your baby's name into their system, reducing (in theory) the hassle over payments for your newborn's health care.

Equally important, you and your partner should have life and disability insurance so your child can be cared for should you die or become disabled. If either of you already have life insurance, update your beneficiaries to include the baby after he's born. While no one likes to think about dying, when you have a child, you must plan for the possibility that you'll die before he's grown. Denial won't pay the bills; life insurance might.

In the United States, 2014 brings the first wave of changes mandated by the 2010 Affordable Care Act (ACA), also known as Obamacare. Under the ACA, a health-insurance company can't deny coverage to anyone based on a "pre-existing condition," such as problems in a pregnancy. Meanwhile, the separate states are supposed to implement health insurance "exchanges" to help individuals for whom coverage is too expensive.

The full impact of the ACA will take several years to determine, in part because regulations are still rolling out and in part because for-profit companies provide most health insurance policies—a system unlike other industrialized countries. However, there are some encouraging initial signs. For instance, many state insurance exchanges are turning out to be less expensive than policy makers (and Obamacare critics) feared. If you don't have health insurance through your employer, you'll want to get coverage through your state's insurance exchange.

The U.S. Department of Health and Human Services oversees the ACA guidelines and implementation. You can learn more about the ACA and insurance in general at healthcare.gov.

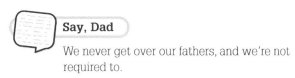

Say, Dad

We never get over our fathers, and we're not required to.

—Irish Proverb

If you live in Canada, your health-care road may have some bumps, but universal health care guarantees you aren't thrown into a ditch for lack of money.

Making Out Your Will

Dwelling on the subject of death is no fun, even though it happens to all of us. Nevertheless, now that you'll be parents, you and your partner should have wills. A will is simply a legal document that tells how to distribute your assets and care for any children you have after your death.

If you have a will already, update it now to account for the fact that you're becoming a father. Otherwise, some probate judge you've never met will make all those decisions for you—not smart and very preventable.

An essential piece of information you and your partner should include in your wills is the name of the guardian you choose to care for your child if you aren't around. If just one of you dies, the surviving parent usually takes the role of guardian. Outside of you and your partner, a guardian must be an adult who's willing to take on the task. Don't name someone until you've discussed it with them—and they've agreed to do it. Most parents choose a relative who shares the parents' values and beliefs about child-rearing and (most important) will love, comfort, and nurture the child.

Your will also lays out how you want your assets—money, real estate, and so on—distributed upon your death and who you want to oversee the management of the will (an executor).

You can find forms to make a simple will online, in books, or at the library. However, when children are involved, it pays to create your will with the help of an attorney. Estate and probate law (the area covering postdeath decisions) varies from state to state, sometimes substantially. If you don't already have a lawyer, ask for references for a lawyer in your area who specializes in this type of law.

Saving for College

The first day of college for your child is a long time off, but it will also be a lot more expensive than it already is now. For the last 30 years, college tuition costs have been rising at rates far beyond the average rate of inflation. It's difficult to get an accurate estimate of what a school will cost 18 years from now, but there are no signs of tuition and fees leveling off. Therefore, now is a good time to start thinking about what you want to do to save for your child's education.

Some parents decide to invest a set percentage of their income for college, starting when their babies are little. If this is what you'd like to do, it's best to use a financial planner to decide what saving tools (savings bonds, mutual funds, and so on) will work best for your situation and goals.

One option in the United States is a 529 College Savings Plan (named after Section 529 of the Internal Revenue Code), which has assets free from federal income tax. There are two types of 529 plans: prepaid tuition plans and college savings plans. Most states offer only one or the other type of plan, and a few offer both.

With a prepaid tuition plan, the state guarantees your child will be able to attend an in-state public college at rates effectively equivalent to today's tuition rate in 18 years. Your principal is at little if any risk, making it a great option financially; however, this plan limits your flexibility, since you must reside in the state and you make up the difference if your child decides on a private or out-of-state school.

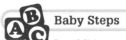 **Baby Steps**

In addition to state-sponsored 529 plans, a consortium of more than 270 private colleges and universities offer an independent "prepaid tuition" 529 plan. For more information, see privatecollege529.com.

A college savings plan operates more like a traditional IRA. The fund is tax-exempt, but there are no guarantees for how much its value will grow or whether there will be enough money to pay for your child's college expenses when the time comes. However, your child will retain the flexibility to choose a college without being limited to in-state institutions.

Anyone (for example, grandparents) can contribute to a 529 plan, but there are regulations that prevent people from "hiding" investments beyond what's needed to pay for the child's education. For more information about the 529 plans and other financial aid, check out Federal Student Aid, an office of the U.S. Department of Education, at studentaid.ed.gov/.

The Canadian government offers a similar tool, called registered education savings plans (RESPs), that grow tax free until the child is ready for university, college, or a vocational institute. RESP contributions up to $2,500 per year are eligible for a 20 percent Canada Education Savings Grant, up to a lifetime maximum grant of $7,200 per child. An additional grant is available for low- and middle-income families; however, you'd need to file a separate application needs to receive it.

You can find more information about your RESP options from CanLearn at canlearn.ca/eng/savings/know_your_resp.shtml.

Your Work Path

Your new baby will affect your career and work life, even though most of the attention goes to how it will affect your partner's employment. Because pregnancy allows more time for clear thinking than midnight feedings do, now is when you should start planning your work path.

Your partner's pregnancy is a perfect period to examine your instincts, assumptions, and expectations about your role as a father. You may initially think you'll have to work longer and harder at your job because you'll need more money for your baby. On the other hand, your first instinct may be that you'll have to cut back on paid work so you'll be free to spend lots of time with the baby. Or you may feel whipsawed between these and other scenarios.

No matter what you do, keep your mind and heart open to the possibilities for work-life balance.

What Is a WFBP?

Through polls, research, and even your friends and other family members, you may see a wide spectrum of work-life situations. But how are you going to create a workable path through you own specific work and family situation?

Your best bet is to write down a work-family balance plan (WFBP). Why get it on paper? Because you can't successfully balance work and fathering on the fly. You'll certainly fly by the seat of your pants on occasion, but having a plan will help minimize those occasions.

 Say, Dad

What's a good investment? Go home from work early and spend the afternoon throwing a ball around with your son.

—Ben Stein, actor and political commentator

Just as with a birth plan, a good WFBP is a flexible work in progress. Start by brainstorming what you want to have happen in your life once the baby comes, such as aspirations, hopes, dreams, career advancement, and education. Once you have that list written down, talk with your partner, trusted friends, and other family members about what they need and value the most from a good parent. With that information to guide you, prioritize the list you brainstormed to make your WFBP.

In your WFBP, write down ways you can be more productive at work and at home. Think about how you'll manage your time between both places, keeping in mind you'll need to adjust your expectations as you go along.

For your life outside of work, build in time for exercise, nurturing the relationship with your partner, being with extended family, and having fun. Also, think about scheduling regular "you-and-me" time with the baby. Let's say you get home from work at 6:00 and your baby's bedtime is 7:00—you can make it your routine to take the baby on a "wind-down-and-relax" walk; read him a story; or otherwise be a familiar, influential, everyday presence in his life.

As for your work life, set expectations for yourself and your workplace, such as shortening your commute or taking time off to be with your baby. Don't be afraid to use your work's family leave time. Many companies offer time off for new parents to bond with their infants. Unfortunately, in most cases, the leave is unpaid—and only taken by mothers. You and your baby need and deserve family leave, too. After all, family emergencies aren't the only legitimate excuse for leaving work to be a father.

When filling out your WFBP, remember: don't substitute money for time. You need to provide financially, but not at the expense of providing your presence and yourself to your family.

 Attention, Please

If reflection and planning lead you to the conclusion that your current job isn't able to give you the amount of time you want with your family, set a strategy for finding a new one. To do this, follow father Jeremy Adam Smith's advice: Find yourself a family-friendly workplace, and decide how much money that's worth to you.

You can read more of Smith's tips at greatergood.berkeley.edu/article/item/ how_to_be_a_happy_working_dad.

When you've completed a first draft of your WFBP, review it with your partner and trusted friends for their perspectives and advice. You can also write up a version of your plan and share it with your boss. This may help her feel involved in your process, increasing the chances that she will get on board with the plan.

Keep referring to your plan and use it as your guide to being a worker among workers and a dad among dads. If you divert from the plan, that's okay. You'll never achieve perfection with your plan or how you execute it. Commit to it anyway.

If you need more ideas for a WFBP, check out fatherhood.org/ fathers/articles/new-dads/work-family-balance/plan-for-balance.

Family Time Now

Men who care for their children still face discrimination in the workplace. Recent research from the University of Toronto and University of Long Island-Post finds that middle-class men in non-traditional caregiving roles are treated worse at work than men who retain traditional gender norms in the family. And as Dr. Jennifer Berdahl of Toronto's Rotman School of Management discussed in an issue of *Science Daily,* "Their hours are no different than other employees', but their co-workers appear to be picking up on their non-traditional caregiving roles and are treating them disrespectfully."

For the most part, family, friends, employers, and others will simply assume that your partner will need to cut back on employment to care for the new baby. Despite improving attitudes about fathers, few people will think twice (if they even think once) about the "Mom – Work = Kids" mindset; instead, they'll assume you won't need to adjust your schedule very much for your partner's pregnancy and your baby's arrival.

You may have to challenge some of these assumptions inside yourself, as well as with others. As you do, you'll need to work at getting on people's radar as a "primary parent" who needs support and understanding to maintain your obligation to family and workplace.

 Say, Dad

There's nothing better than excelling at a game you love. There's nothing worse than thinking your accomplishments as a player outweigh your responsibilities as a person.

—Doug Flutie, football player

Start out by talking honestly with your boss (or, if you're self-employed, your clients/customers) about the pregnancy. A direct approach helps establish an expectation that you're committed to being a full parenting partner now and after your baby's birth.

At the same time, the pregnancy gives you the opportunity to demonstrate you're able and willing to continue handling responsibilities on your work team, even while taking time away from the workplace for doctors' appointments with your partner. The pregnancy months also give you time to find solutions for concerns and unanticipated problems at work. This kind of time management shows your boss and colleagues you can juggle fatherhood and career. It also lays a foundation of trust in your ability, commitment, and judgment on the job and at home.

And who knows? By taking these steps, you may also help break down barriers for current and future colleagues and fathers who want to commit to both work and parenting.

The Stay-At-Home Dad Option

Can a new father be the parent who cares for the baby full time? That may sound like a radical (or radically silly) question; nevertheless, the number of stay-at-home fathers is growing steadily.

Some men do it because they instinctively feel well suited or called to the task. Some do it because they're unemployed. A dad may even stay home because his partner has the higher salary and his income wouldn't cover the cost of professional day care. And while most stay-at-home dads (self-described as SAHDs, even though the job is a lot of fun) re-enter the paid workforce once their children enter school, a few remain "primary parent" for years beyond.

If the SAHD life sounds appealing, don't let other people's confusion, suspicion, or resistance deter you. Feel free to challenge dismissive attitudes expressed in belittling comments like "Hi there, Mr. Mom!" (As if anyone calls a female parent Mrs. Dad or even Mrs. Mom.)

The U.S. Census reports that there are now about 189,000 stay-at-home dads, caring for 369,000 children—a clear sign that SAHDs aren't freaks of nature. As for the "Mr. Mom" stereotype, daddy blogger Chris Bernholdt (dadncharge.com) says, "I wouldn't base my knowledge of Australia on what I have seen in 'Crocodile Dundee,' so why would anyone keep using a reference from a 30-year-old film that is also sexist?"

Being a SAHD has many benefits for you and your family. Longitudinal research by Yale psychiatrist Kyle Pruitt, MD, and others indicates that SAHDs have stronger bonds with their children than other fathers (another commonsense example of how quantity facilitates quality). In addition, the children with SAHDs seem to have more confidence and a stronger sense of self. Studies also suggest that working mothers are more involved in their children's lives when the father stays at home when compared to families who use professional day care.

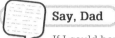

Say, Dad

If I could have one wish for my own sons, it is that they should have the courage of women.

—Adrienne Rich, poet

Beginning in 1980, I had the amazing good fortune to be an at-home dad for much of my daughters' childhood. I continued to work, but often part time and at odd hours; for example, I spent years doing morning radio with a workday that went from 4 A.M. to noon, leaving the rest of the day for being with the kids.

This wasn't always easy. Part-time work meant part-time pay, so my family had a very tight budget. Working odd hours also meant being sleep-deprived frequently. On reflection, however, I realized other dads battled those problems no matter how they spent their daylight hours!

Perhaps my biggest struggle was overcoming the deeply internalized notion that I was failing as a father because I wasn't making more money or getting promotions. It took years before I could fully believe that providing my time and attention was providing more value to my family than a fatter paycheck.

Some folks are surprised by how close my daughters and I were and still are now that they're adults. However, no one in our family is surprised. Family members (and other AHDs) understand how it works. Be around and responsible for your kids from diaper days to the first driving lesson, and you get to know and love each other very well. You also manage to drive each other crazy sometimes, but that's family.

So give the at-home option serious consideration; the payoff can be huge. No, my retirement plan isn't as hefty as some other middle-aged men I know, but my father-child affection account is about as full as it can get.

If you'd like more information on being an AHD, check out the website athomedad.org. It has the best collection of resources on common AHD issues, such as starting a playgroup with other dads, running a home business, dealing with personal problems (divorce, death, custody, bias, and so on), and networking with other AHDs.

The Least You Need to Know

- Understand the legal and other implications of having a child when married, unmarried, or in a same-sex couple.
- Get your financial house in order before the baby comes by working out a family budget, getting health insurance, and updating your will.
- Plan your work-family balance now, so you'll be investing your time and energy where they need to be most after your baby arrives.

PART 4

Turning the Corner

You've learned a lot and laid some plans over the course of this pregnancy. Now it's time to know what happens right before, during, and after your baby is born.

This part gives you information, guidance, and additional planning tools to help you be a first-rate birth coach who's prepared to help your partner through labor and delivery.

You also learn how to bring your baby safely back to a loving home, where you play a key role. This parts shows you how to build your bond with your child from day one through holding, feeding, soothing, burping, changing diapers, playing, and putting the baby to sleep.

Finally, you learn how to create a vision of the father you hope and want to be. You're about to traverse the mysterious divide between expecting to be and actually being a dad. Get ready for the ride of your life!

CHAPTER 10

Ready to Launch: Planning for the Big Day

In This Chapter

- Developing a birth plan
- Preparing transportation and supplies
- Recognizing the signs of labor
- Taking care of the paperwork

To be ready for the exciting day your baby is born, you should invest time now in planning what to do when labor starts, what supplies you and your partner will need, and how to get to the hospital or birthing center. You also need to know what the signs are that it's time for the baby to come.

In this chapter, I go over what you can do to get ready both for your partner going into labor and for what happens when you first get to the hospital.

Making Preparations

When your partner finally goes into labor, your adrenaline will start pumping overtime. All the anticipatory nerves, worries, and excitement may send your mind spinning as you race to the hospital—perhaps without your phone and house keys. Therefore, unless you regularly display superhuman calm and clear thinking in a crisis (and even if you do), make sure you plan ahead. You and your partner need to take the time to think through what you both want or need to happen on the day of your baby's birth.

Making a Birth Plan

Most expectant parents write up a birth plan—a document stating what you want and expect to happen during your pregnancy, labor, and delivery. A birth plan gives you a role in planning and helps you be explicit about your wishes with each other and with the doctor.

 Pregnant Pause

You may not get every wish on your list if health insurance doesn't cover a service you want or the hospital doesn't provide it. Your doctor or midwife may also have opinions on the risks and benefits of any options you propose. Keep an open mind as you discuss your plan with them.

Many OB/GYNs, midwives, and hospitals offer birth plan forms or templates to help you along. You may also have to fill out additional forms or releases ahead of time for certain options. Here's the sort of information the birth plan should contain:

* Medical problems during pregnancy (diabetes, STDs, anemia, and so on)

* What type of birth you are planning

* Who else (if anyone) you want to be in the room during labor and delivery

* The atmosphere you want to have in the room during labor and delivery

- Whether your partner wants to stand up, lie down, use a shower, or walk around during labor

- Whether you want fetal monitoring

- Your preferences on inducing labor

- What type of pain relief (if any) your partner wants

- The physical position she wants to be in during delivery

- Your feelings about using a forceps or vacuum assistance during delivery

- Your feelings about episiotomy

- Whether you want to cut the umbilical cord, save the cord blood, or donate it

- What happens if you need a C-section

- If your partner wants to breastfeed and when she wants to start

A birth plan can also lay out your wishes for the first hours of your newborn's life, giving the hospital staff important guidance on the following:

- Medical exams or tests

- Using a pacifier

- Giving your baby vitamins

- Your baby's first bath

- Feeding preferences, such as whether to use formula

- Circumcision if you have a boy

If you can't find a template through your doctor or would like another option, check out the birth plan worksheet at assets.baby-center.com/ims/Content/birthplan_pdf.pdf.

Remember that your birth plan is a work in progress. Review it with the doctor and your partner. In addition, consider asking veteran parents about their labor and delivery stories. These points of view can help guide you in planning.

Attention, Please

There's no guarantee that a breech baby won't poke a big hole in your quiet, incense-laden plans for the birth. In the end, the first priority is always the safety and health of the baby and mother.

You don't need to have strong feelings about any particular element of the plan, and it's okay to change your mind. In fact, it's important for you to stay flexible because you may need to change parts of your birth plan.

Make sure you deliver a complete copy to your doctor and the hospital or birthing center, and tell them to attach it to your partner's medical record. Make sure you have a copy, too, and bring it with you when your partner goes into labor. That way, if you go into labor while your doctor is out of town or off duty, you can just give the birth plan to the doctor who does attend you (it may also be in your partner's medical records), and he'll have a concrete guide to your approach. Simply put, a birth plan is worth the effort.

Arranging Transportation

You can take simple (if a bit time-consuming) steps to prepare for getting from your home to the hospital or birthing center when the big moment comes.

First off, put the phone numbers for your doctor and hospital (or birthing center) on the refrigerator or some other easy-to-find location in your home. When labor starts, you may not have the time and attention to search for it on your phone, on the internet, or in the junk drawer. Put a copy of the phone numbers in the glove compartment of your car, too, since you may not be at home when labor begins.

If you plan to be the driver, take some practice trips from home to the hospital one or two months before the due date in order to find (and memorize) the best route. Make sure you also check online to see if any government agencies plan to start construction projects along your chosen path around the time of your partner's due date, so you can allow for detours and traffic delays.

Whatever route you decide to take, try driving it during the worst of the morning and evening rush hours, so the "worst-case scenario" data is in your planning. Factor in the climate and weather, too. For instance, I lived for many years in Duluth, Minnesota. (Spoiler alert: it snows a lot there.) Early on, I learned a good tip for driving in the middle of a snowstorm: follow the city busses; their routes always get plowed first.

By the middle of the third trimester, your vehicle should be saddled up and ready to run on a moment's notice. Get the oil changed, top off the tank frequently, and check the tires. If it's winter and you live in Duluth (or its climatic equivalent), make sure the battery will start in the middle of a subzero night. And install the infant car safety seat in your vehicle at least a month before your partner's due date. You'll need it to bring baby home, and you can save a trip by setting it up now!

Attention, Please

Keep an extra set of car and house keys in plain sight—ideally, next to the doctor's phone number or on a hook in a spot you pass on the way out the door to your vehicle. This can save you search-and-scramble time in a pinch.

For safety's sake, line up a substitute driver or two who can step (or drive) in during an emergency—ideally, it should be someone who lives close by. Make sure they have easy access to their own vehicle and to yours, and give them a set of car and house keys for the duration. That way, if your partner goes into labor and you're stuck somewhere away from home, you won't have to manage backup logistics over the phone.

If you and your partner live without your own vehicles, work out logistics best suited for your situation:

* **Ambulance:** This is the most expensive option, but it can also be the most necessary if your partner is having problems, it's unsafe to drive, or other emergencies arise. Call 911 to summon one.

- **Buddy ride:** Ask a vehicle-owning friend (or two) to be available to drive you and your partner. Make sure the person lives close, is willing to drive in the middle of the night, and doesn't fall right back to sleep after you call him!

- **Public transit:** Get current schedules and keep them accessible. "Preride" the bus or subway route during different times of day, so you know how long the trip will take. Also, keep the exact fare and extra public transit cards where you can see—and grab—them on the way out the door.

- **Taxi:** Call one or more cab companies to ask how long it normally takes to reach your address during rush hour, at 2 in the morning, and so on. Make sure you also get an estimate of the fare from your place to the hospital—and ask whether the cabbies take credit cards. It's a good idea to keep the taxi company's phone number next to the doctor's phone number and program it into your phone so it's easy to access when you need it. And don't forget to keep enough cash for the fare someplace where you'll know where it is when in a rush.

Preparing a Bag

Your partner may be in the hospital for a few hours or for several days—you can't know for sure. Therefore, you should prepare a bag of supplies she will need for labor, delivery, and perhaps a longer stay ahead of time. And because you'll be in the hospital during labor, delivery, and the aftermath, you'll need a few things, too.

Start by making a list of things you and your partner will need to stay focused and feel as comfortable as possible during labor. Here are some ideas to get you started:

- A toothbrush, toothpaste, hairbrush, and other essential toiletries

- Medications and vitamins

- Eyeglasses or contacts and supplies (bring an extra pair just in case)

- A night gown and robe for your partner to wear, if the hospital will allow it

- Slippers and warm socks

- Several pairs of *cotton* underwear; cotton will be more breathable and comfortable for her

- A list of names and phone numbers for people you'll want to call to share your news, in case you're unable to use your cell phone in the hospital or your cell battery goes dead

- A book or magazine to distract both of you

- A camera, camcorder, and so on with fresh batteries, a charger, and film (if you're old-fashioned enough to know what film is)

- Headphones and an MP3 player, if your partner likes listening to music—you two can compile a playlist now, so you're ready with relaxing, energizing, celebratory, or other tune types you'll want during and after labor

- Comfortable clothes and shoes for your partner to wear home

- Sweatpants and a T-shirt or other comfortable clothes for you to sleep in; the people you don't know in the hospital (in other words, most of them) will appreciate a little modesty

- Low-odor, high-energy snacks to keep up *your* energy level during labor, and an extra "victory" snack for her eat after the delivery

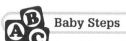 **Baby Steps**

A bathing suit lets you join your partner in the shower to relax during labor. You'll also need one if you're using a birthing tub.

The bag should not include items that would cause you big problems if you lost them on your way to the hospital, while you're there, or on the way home, such as the following:

- Jewelry and other personally valuable items

- Credit cards

- Extra cameras, tablets, phones, or other electronic gear

- Excess amounts of cash

You don't have to pack much for the baby, since the hospital will have diapers and simple clothes to cover her. However, you'll need a "onesie" or sleeper, socks (no shoes until your baby is walking!), and receiving blankets (infant-sized, lightweight blankets). Many parents also like to have a special outfit for the baby's trip home or for "showing-off" hours in the hospital.

Do your best to confine the materials to one bag, minimizing how much you have to carry from the house to the vehicle, the vehicle into the hospital, and to multiple locations within the hospital. If an unanticipated circumstance arises after you're already inside the hospital, have a relative or friend go to your house and retrieve any additional things you need.

And don't worry if your birth bag isn't within easy reach when you head to the hospital. If she goes into labor at the mall, head straight to the ER; don't stop home for the bag (or anything else) beforehand. Believe me, your partner can give birth successfully without extra socks.

Time to Go!

From the moment you two learned you were pregnant, you've probably wondered, "How do we know when to head to the hospital?" Your OB/GYN and childbirth classes provide some guidance on what to look for and how to know it's time to go. However, you must make sure you understand the stages and phases of labor and delivery, as well as what's required of you in terms of information when you first get to the hospital.

Labor Breakdown

Medical professionals break down labor and delivery into three stages:

* **Stage 1, phase 1:** Relatively mild contractions which start dilating the cervix to 3 centimeters (out of 10).

* **Stage 1, phase 2:** Contractions continue and intensify, dilating the cervix up to 7 centimeters.

* **Stage 1, phase 3:** The cervix dilates completely to 10 centimeters, which means the baby's path is ready for delivery.

* **Stage 2:** The mom finally starts pushing to deliver the baby.

* **Stage 3:** The mom delivers the placenta.

In this chapter, I focus on the first two phases of stage 1, because they usually happen at home. By the time your partner is transitioning to stage 1, phase 3, the contractions are stronger, her cervix is nearing full dilation, and you need to be at the hospital or birthing center (see Chapter 11 for more on stages 2 and 3).

True or False?

Your first challenge is likely to be determining whether your partner's contractions are the beginnings of stage 1 or are Braxton-Hicks contractions. Braxton-Hicks contractions are what many people call "false" labor. False labor can start early in the third trimester and reappear until real labor begins.

How can you tell the difference? Braxton-Hicks contractions will be like the following:

* Uncomfortable (like menstrual discomfort) rather than featuring sharp pain

* Not rhythmic

* Infrequent and irregular

* Unlikely to grow in intensity as they continue

* Likely to fade away after a couple minutes or less

Braxton-Hicks contractions may also cease when your partner moves around or changes her body position—the real ones don't. You can provide some relief from Braxton-Hicks contractions if you bring her water or a snack, take her for a walk, or encourage a nap.

And don't worry about Braxton-Hicks contractions harming your baby. According to University of North Dakota's Joy Dorscher, MD, Braxton-Hicks contractions are more like "practice runs" to help get your partner, her uterus, and the baby ready for actual contractions.

As for when the real deal begins, stage 1, phase 1 contractions occur every 10 minutes and with a frequency of at or above five times an hour. During this phase of contractions, your partner will feel new pressure on her pelvis or vagina.

The pain will start in her back and move to her abdomen—or vice versa—and the contractions will steadily increase in strength. If your partner walks around or shifts positions and the contractions keep coming, that's a clue they're actual contractions and not Braxton-Hicks contractions. Feeling nauseous, vomiting, or having diarrhea can also be signs that stage 1, phase 1 has started.

As soon as you suspect that genuine stage 1 labor has begun, start timing the length of each contraction, along with the amount of time between the end of one contraction and the start of the next. Then call the doctor or hospital and explain your partner's symptoms. They'll ask you (or her) some questions to help determine where she is in the process. They'll also tell you whether to head to the hospital now.

By the time your partner is transitioning from stage 1, phase 2, to stage 1, phase 3, you should be at the hospital (or at least on your way there), because she's entering the most intense part of labor.

If you see vaginal bleeding or any fluid coming out of the vagina, call the doctor. And get moving if her amniotic sac has ruptured (a.k.a. her water breaks). That means the baby no longer has the protection of the sac, and a physician has to decide on what steps to take, such as inducing labor.

Filling Out Paperwork

When you arrive at the hospital, you have to complete some forms. Have you ever entered the doors of any large institutions that *didn't* require you to fill out paperwork?

Medical staff will start testing and monitoring your partner and the baby as soon as you arrive. This "triage" procedure helps them determine how imminent delivery may be or whether there are immediate problems with the childbirth. In most cases, this leaves you in charge of the paper. If your partner is whisked off while you're handling admission forms, find out the following:

- Where they are taking her

- Where she will be after you're done filling out forms

- Whether you can defer some or all of the paperwork until after you've helped your partner settle in and you get a better handle on where you are in the labor process

Make sure you're already carrying your health insurance cards and identification at all times, as you'll need those right away at the hospital.

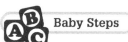

Baby Steps

A growing number of hospitals and birthing centers allow you and your partner to fill out some forms weeks ahead of time. This may reduce—but not eliminate—the info you must provide and papers you must sign upon your arrival.

The hospital will want proof of insurance, contact information for you, the name of your physician, and so on. You may also need to sign release forms to give permission for the facility to treat your partner, take tests, and provide other services. If you have questions or are unsure about the information they're seeking, arrange to provide the material later, after the birth.

You may also need some determination if you're not married and encounter resistance about your role, responsibilities, and access from any staff. Be patient (yelling only increases resistance) while asserting your place and your voice.

The Least You Need to Know

- Complete your birth plan early, so you can examine its feasibility and have it ready to use on short notice.
- Take the logistical lead for planning the trip from home to the hospital.
- The beginning of labor and Braxton-Hicks contractions feel very different, so learn the signs of genuine versus "false" labor.
- Start managing your partner's care as soon as you go through the hospital door by handling the paperwork.

Delivery Day

In This Chapter

- Smartly sharing the news of what's happening
- Supporting your partner through the stages of labor
- Being a part of your baby's delivery
- Delivering the baby yourself in an emergency

Childbirth is a life-changing moment that burns into a father's memory. My most vivid memory of the day my twin daughters were born is seeing each of them come out—actual, individual people right from the start. I also remember the surroundings of the delivery room in great detail—much more intensely than normal for such a short span of moments (even though it didn't feel short at the time). You'll soon experience such images, moments, and memories for yourself.

Whether labor and delivery go swiftly or slowly, you need to know what to do and when. This chapter guides you through a brief and miraculous moment in your life: your child's birth day.

Words to the Wise

Like most expectant dads, you may worry about how you'll react during labor and delivery. Common anxieties include the following:

- What if my coaching isn't good enough to support her?

- I'm afraid I'll make mistakes.

- Is she going to scream and curse at me?

- Will I get too exhausted to be any help?

- Will I have enough energy, concentration, and focus to do what needs doing?

- How will I keep track of what the doctors and nurses are telling me and what they're doing?

- I've never done this before. It's a total mystery and I don't really know what it's going to be like!

These are completely normal fears to have. Fortunately, our species has developed amazing capacities in fathers that can help you deal with the situation (and your anxieties).

When you're in the middle of labor and delivery, you're likely to find sources of energy that you didn't know you had. You may not be fully conscious of it in the moment, but you'll probably have all the concentration, attention, and focus that you and your partner need. Reflecting on labor and delivery, many new dads say things like, "When I think of how tired I was then, I can't believe I made it all the way through" or "I found myself willing to make mistakes, be imperfect, and trust my wife's intuition and trust in her own body."

Just know you're capable of fulfilling your role, and by the end of delivery day, you and your partner will have a very special child (or children) of your own.

Taking Your Own Tweet Time

Updating your online status may be second nature for you. Perhaps you tweet and post everyday occurrences in real time without a second thought. However, pregnancy, labor, and delivery aren't ordinary events, so posting updates on every stage of your baby's birth isn't always the best strategy.

Well before you're in the hospital, give some thought to how your baby's birth isn't a commonplace part of life. If you decide to use social media during this time, make sure you and your partner have a plan for when to use it. For example, it's counterproductive to let social media disrupt your focus and intensity during labor and delivery. Being present and attentive with your partner and new-born is far more important than how long your Twitter followers wait before they get word of the baby's arrival.

Also, recognize that one or both of you may be exhausted or otherwise in an altered psychological state during labor. If you decide to use social media, use discretion; you don't want to "Tumbl" into hard feelings when spreading the word online. Here are some ways you and your partner can control the flow of information:

* Give each other review and "veto" power over any messages you want to send.

* Keep updates simple. What seems clever and witty during the intensity of labor may not translate well to others.

* Tell your closest relatives and friends about major developments (*especially* the birth itself) before informing your wide circle of followers.

* Use your mobile device as a telephone and call your parents, siblings, and grandparents to share the good news. They want to hear the enthusiasm in your voice, and you'll love hearing their excitement and pride.

You also need to decide beforehand whether and when to accept phone calls or messages from family and friends while your partner is in labor. Other people will be eager for updates, but you get to decide if you have the time and bandwidth to respond.

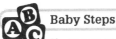 **Baby Steps**

If you want to keep in touch with others via social media or other ways during the labor and delivery, it's smart to have a backup plan. Bring a printout with phone numbers, usernames, and passwords with you to the hospital.

Above all, check to see whether the hospital or birthing center allows cell phones. Some facilities still have bans on cell phone use inside the building, meaning the staff will have you shut down your smartphone. Also, it's difficult to get reception in many hospitals, with their large structures and loads of electronic equipment. To contact others, you may have to go outside the building to make calls on your phone or use a payphone. (Google "phone booth" if you've never seen one!)

Labor Continues

Most pregnant women get to the hospital in the final phase of labor's first stage (see Chapter 10 for stage 1's early phases). You won't necessarily see a clear demarcation line between stage 1 and stage 2. However, you'll know you're getting much closer to delivery when the contractions are more intense and come closer together. Your partner is now about to pass through the arduous process that ultimately leads to childbirth.

She's likely to need all of her concentration to get through each contraction, so take the lead in timing the contractions' length and intervals. The more she's concentrating, the shorter and simpler your communication should be. Keep your voice loving, not snappish, and avoid disputes or lengthy explanations. Regardless of what happens during labor, you need to present your partner with an upbeat, comforting, and encouraging face.

 Attention, Please

Two brave (or naïve) fathers tried to replicate labor pains in their own bodies. Watch the results in this video: youtu.be/qtR_-MINR1o. Perhaps they're both brave *and* naïve!

As stage 2 progresses, your partner may get the urge to start pushing the baby out. Many moms say the urge seems impossible to resist. However, she shouldn't push until your doctor gives the green light. You may have to spend several minutes (or longer) helping her to resist that urge until the time is right.

Meanwhile, relax—really! Take a deep breath, roll your shoulders, stretch your joints, and keep your focus.

"The Wait"

Don't expect your partner to have a "normal" labor—there's no such thing. Some labors (even a few first-time ones) last an hour, while others can last days. A first-time mother tends to have longer labor, since it's her body's first attempt to pull off this incredible feat. Therefore, resist the temptation to have a "schedule," even unconsciously. Labor will take how long it takes. There may be long stretches between intense contractions, short stretches between weaker contractions, short stretches between intense contractions … you get the idea.

This experience isn't a debate, subject to parliamentary procedure. For people in an intimate relationship, especially under duress, logic doesn't work—but love does. No matter what she says or doesn't say, demonstrate your love and caring.

One way to help her is to handle only one contraction at a time. Don't worry about the next one in the middle of the current one, and don't criticize her or how she's doing things. Act the way you would want her to act if she was helping you through hours of intense pain. If encouraging words make her tense, then encourage and reassure silently with your eyes and touch.

You can also start using the tools from childbirth classes to get her through. For example, if you learned Lamaze, do the breathing and focusing with her. At the same time, be open to spontaneous adjustments. Let's say you practiced your breathing while holding hands. She may want to hold hands during her labor breathing, or she may not, as some women feel irritated when another person touches their skin during labor. Follow her lead, realizing that her desires and needs may change abruptly a few minutes from now.

Contractions are very draining, and she needs energy when it comes time to push the baby down the birth canal. Therefore, do everything you can to help her relax so she doesn't burn through energy needlessly.

If you're concerned about how things are progressing, ask the doctor or nurses. They're used to these questions, and you (or your insurer) are paying them to help you.

In a complication-free labor, outpourings of oxytocin help trigger contractions in the mother's body. If that doesn't happen and labor slows down too much, the doctor is likely to suggest "inducing" labor. That usually means giving the mother a synthetic oxytocin drug through an IV. (The most common brand names are Pitocin and Syntocinon.) This medication can have unpleasant side effects— such as nausea, vomiting, sinus pain, and memory problems—but the drug also causes more severe and frequent contractions, so the labor can continue to progress.

 Attention, Please

Labor doesn't always go according to plan. For example, when my daughter was in labor, my grandson's head came down on one side of her cervix and stayed there. The cervix got swollen, complicating things (and generating lots of pain), even while the cervix dilated. This was just one of the wrinkles in a 34-hour labor, during which Mom and Dad showed incredible patience and courage.

Whatever You Want, Baby

From the moment you enter the hospital, you are your partner's hard drive, advocate, and translator. In mid-contraction, she's unlikely to remember much (or anything) that a nurse or doctor tells her. Work to retain the medical information and suggestions, repeating them to her if necessary. In addition, keep the staff aware of your presence without being annoying. Find people to answer questions when you have them. If the doctor hasn't checked on your partner lately, go out in the hall and request a visit.

Your partner may be too tired or distracted to speak up for what she needs and wants. You know her better than the medical staff anyway, so advocate for her. For example, if there's no emergency, insist you two be given time to consider treatment options before moving ahead with a procedure. And because you'll have more mental bandwidth during this time, work as the go-between for her and the doctors and staff. Relay any questions or answers from the staff to your partner promptly and calmly in a way she can easily comprehend.

This is also a time to ease your partner's physical discomfort in whatever ways you can. Because the contractions are now longer and more painful, your partner is turning her attention completely to her body and what's happening to it. She'll have more of the vaginal discharge known as "bloody show," along with aching legs, growing fatigue, and backache. If she's never been in labor before, she won't know for sure how to get physical relief. Encourage her to "listen" to her body and follow her intuition (remembering that nature knows how to help the process along). You can suggest standing up, lying down, walking, showering, watching TV, or massaging her back or feet. When making suggestions, keep from having an agenda; if she turns down your offer, don't assume you know best and insist she go along.

Traditionally, one of the roles of the father was feeding the mother a steady supply of ice chips to relieve her thirst. That's because doctors didn't want much (or anything) in the mother's stomach in case she needed general anesthesia for a C-section. Within the last five years, however, the American College of Obstetricians and Gynecologists issued new guidelines saying that, if the labor has no complication, it's safe for a woman to drink clear liquids like water, sports drinks, herbal tea, and clear broth. Your partner can also have something cold, such as a juice pop. Be forewarned, however: some women do vomit during labor. As Leslie Kardos, MD, chief of gynecology at the California Pacific Medical Center in San Francisco, puts it, "You don't want to eat or drink anything you don't want to see again."

Another way you can bring her relief is by putting a cool, damp washcloth on her neck, forehead, wrists, or other spots. However, wring out the cloth well so you can avoid leaving her skin uncomfortably wet or clammy. And make sure you're prepared with a blanket and socks if she gets a chill afterward.

 Pregnant Pause

If your "let me comfort you" efforts annoy her, back off without backing away. Reassure her you're still there, ready to help in any way you can. And be patient— something that bugged her a half hour ago may be exactly what she wants right now.

Discretion, or How to Avoid Getting Punched

As your partner is having contractions, make sure to keep your focus on getting her through each one and on to the delivery room. During her most painful moments, your partner may shout, "Why did you do this to me? I'm never letting you touch me again! Get lost! I'm going home."

Of course, she can't go home and she will sleep with you again (probably). However, her feelings, thoughts, and outbursts stem from the pain, fatigue, fear, confusion, and frustration she's experiencing. It's a lot for her to handle. That means it's a lot for you to handle.

However, as hard as it will feel, don't take any of this personally. Let her zingers roll off you like water off a duck's back. (Remember, during labor, you are better off being a Daddy Duck than a Daffy Duck.) She's in a lot of pain, so this isn't the right atmosphere for couples counseling.

You can also save yourself trouble by using words and phrases that can help your partner. Before the rush of delivery day, take some time to practice and think about positive words and phrases versus problematic ones. For example, during labor, you shouldn't tell your partner you know how she feels. Why not? First, because you don't know, and second, because she will angrily inform you of that fact.

Because you're working to preserve a calm atmosphere, try to avoid triggering anger and tension through what you say.

Here are some other examples of what you shouldn't say to your partner:

* "I'm inviting your boss to come in and watch for a few minutes."

* "Since you just finished a contraction, I'm going out to get some lunch."

* "Can't talk now, I'm checking scores on my phone."

* "When is this gonna be over?"

Different words can convey your empathy and concern with less chance of ticking her off. Try something like the following:

"I [sense, know, see] that you're really [in pain, tired, frustrated]. You've been showing a lot of [courage, determination, stamina] so far, and I [believe, trust, am confident] that you can get through the next [contraction, couple of minutes, medical test]. I [love, worship, admire, respect] you! I can't wait to see our baby!"

It sounds like a confident Mike Krzyzewski in the last two minutes of March Madness, right? That's why they call you the birth coach, so keep her headed toward the goal, even if it feels like you're in the third overtime.

Labor isn't all pain, drama, and excitement, though. You're also likely to go through times when nothing much is happening. Instead of getting bored, seize these moments as a chance for you and your partner to be alone together. This may be the last chance you have for a few weeks (or months).

No matter what happens, you can find comfort in the fact that many women don't remember all the details of labor. In the excitement of meeting their new child, they quickly forget what they said and did. And fortunately, nature helps women forget a lot of labor and delivery—otherwise, they truly would never have sex again!

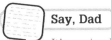

Say, Dad

It's so simple to be wise. Just think of something stupid to say and then don't say it.

—Sam Levenson, author and comedian

So don't let minor complaints or distractions interfere with experiencing this once-in-a-lifetime day. Carpe diem! Or, in this case, "Carpe nativitáte" (seize the birth time)!

The Baby's Coming!

The end of labor approaches quickly as stage 2 speeds along. However, you may feel like you're operating in slow motion. Monumental life events can be like that; your senses sharpen, the events are more vivid, and the memories are more intense.

That's no surprise, since you're about to witness completion of the miraculous process of making a new human being.

Oh, the Pain

At this stage, some contractions may be so intense that she won't be able to even speak during them. Do you have any remaining doubt about the degree of pain your partner feels during labor? Good. Fortunately, this is not news. You and your partner are sharing in something experienced by millions of parents before you.

Modern medicine hasn't eliminated labor pains, but there are some effective ways to ease or mask it:

- Relaxation and concentration practices like Lamaze breathing

- Drugs that block pain in part of the mother's body or (if necessary) knock her out through general anesthesia

You learned about how to help your partner through natural means earlier in this chapter. However, there can be very good reasons to opt for drugs.

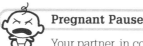

Pregnant Pause

Your partner, in consultation with the doctor, gets to make the pain blocking call. While you may be in great emotional pain watching her in great physical pain, it's not wise to have *your* pain drive the decision.

The following are brief descriptions of the most common anesthetic techniques doctors use during labor:

Epidural block. The doctor or nurse injects anesthesia through the mother's back into an area near the spinal cord called the *epidural*. This requires the doctor to use a long needle and catheter, so you must help your partner remain completely still—even though it hurts.

If successful, an epidural blocks pain in her lower body but lets her stay awake through childbirth. An epidural can sometimes work for a caesarian operation, too. However, if the doctor thinks your partner will deliver within the next hour, she may have to skip this option.

Spinal block. For a spinal block, the needle goes directly into the lower spinal cord. Because the doctor can inject it up until a few moments before delivery, this is considered a last-minute pain option. The side effects of a spinal block last longer than for an epidural.

General anesthesia. This is the full knock-out anesthesia treatment people get for major surgery. Doctors used it routinely for deliveries 50 years ago, but today general anesthesia is rare for a vaginal delivery and can even be avoided in some C-sections.

Pudendal block. If the doctor needs to facilitate delivery with forceps or a suction device, she'll inject a painkiller into the vagina or perineum first. This is less of a production than the preceding options; it's closer to how a dentist numbs your mouth before drilling out a cavity.

Demerol. So-called "narcotic analgesics" such as Demerol are used occasionally during labor, although much less often than decades ago. Just like their cousin morphine, these narcotics can create a range of side effects, such as lightheadedness, dizziness, nausea, vomiting, weakness, headache, agitation, tremors, hallucinations, constipation, disorientation, and sweating.

In addition, your doctor might give your partner or your baby antibiotics to counteract bacteria in the vagina. Babies passing through an infected birth canal have a good chance of catching any local infection, so a course of antibiotics isn't unusual. If there's an active herpes virus, a C-section is the only way to keep the baby from catching it.

Discuss these drugs and the different scenarios in which they can be used at your doctor visits during pregnancy. That way, your doctor will know what pain drug preferences you and your partner have, if any.

Even if you and your partner decide ahead of time to use pain medication, you still need to be flexible and prepared—after all, your baby doesn't know your plan and is operating on his own schedule. If her labor is too far advanced by the time you get to the hospital, the baby may be born before your partner can get any pain meds. Therefore, know all of your options and be ready to use any (or all) of them when delivery day comes. And if she's good at her job, the doctor will remind you and your partner of the need to be flexible both ahead of time and in the hospital.

If you two decide to go completely "natural," remember that a plan is just a plan. Some natural childbirth proponents have zero tolerance for pain-blocking drugs and believe their use means your childbirth isn't natural. This attitude is a bit out of whack. Just because millennia of women gave birth without pharmaceuticals, a drug-free labor and delivery isn't the only "right" childbirth method today.

Say, Dad

My husband complained about his back hurting from standing so long while I was in labor. Bad move, buddy.

—K. C., mother

After all, in the old days, women used folk remedies which altered (if only slightly) the chemistry of their bodies. Plus, many more women and newborns died during childbirth without access to aesthetics and antibiotics—and still do in some parts of the world.

So don't be swayed by someone who tells you using an epidural forfeits the integrity of your labor and delivery. Nature wants your partner and baby to come through childbirth; if that's what happens, with or without drugs, you had a natural childbirth. A good labor and delivery experience demands flexibility.

The (Almost) Final Lap

All of your partner's contractions work to dilate the cervix and widen the path for your baby to travel down the birth canal. Once the cervix is dilated, she's very close to pushing the baby's head out, delivering this new life into your world.

By this point, labor is draining you both and you may wonder whether you can keep it up long enough. In most cases, nature kicks in and finds a way. You may discover you have much deeper supplies of stamina and patience than you imagined.

 Say, Dad

Our labor lasted more than a day, and sometimes when the doctor checked her cervix, it caused unbelievable pain. I'd never seen her in that much pain and it felt almost unbearable. This was definitely the hardest part for me. Then, about midway through, I had a moment when I was aware how much there was a flow to the process, and how in touch she was in her body. It was like she was successfully riding huge waves, and I was incredibly proud of her.

—Mark, father

As the delivery nears, keep coaching your partner through each contraction while listening closely for the doctor's instructions about when and how to push. During these climactic moments, continue to advocate for her and help facilitate communication between her and the doctor.

Witnesses for the Birth

The normal delivery room isn't very crowded. Usually, the birth team includes your partner, the doctor, a nurse or two, and you. But if your medical providers allow it, you can choose to invite others in to witness the birth.

I know a first-time father who was open to the idea of his wife's twin sister attending the birth. "One of those things about marrying a twin," Bob says, "is that they stay close to each other. You have to make room for that."

Fortunately, Bob and his sister-in-law had become good friends, had fairly good boundaries with each other, and had discussed their respective labor and delivery roles well ahead of time. "She understood and accepted that I was the first team for supporting my wife, so we still ended up having an amazing mom-and-dad experience. It was also great to have my wife's twin there to support both of us, and joke with my wife in ways that only twins can. We were all glad we did it together."

If you and your partner want other family members or friends in the delivery room, you should first do the following:

* Discuss the idea with your doctor *before* you extend any invitations.

* Make all of your decisions on who should be there well before your due date.

* Keep the number small. This isn't a wedding, and each additional person more than doubles the potential for communication problems.

* When making the invitation, explicitly state that you and your partner may ask guests to leave the labor or delivery room—and/or ask them for help with tasks and errands—as the situation requires.

* Unless the situation is extraordinary, once you're already at the hospital, don't issue any last-minute invites for family or friends to join you in the labor or delivery room.

* Don't succumb to people demanding that you let them into the room. You and your partner are having a baby, not playing traffic cop. If other people resent your decision, that's their problem.

They key is setting clear boundaries and expectations. If friends or family join you in the labor or delivery room, it's not your job to entertain them. And if, at any moment, you need to ignore them, ask them to be quiet, or tell them to leave, do so without hesitation. After all, they should be there to support you and your partner.

Feeling Queasy?

The actual birth of an infant can include a messy assortment of various sights, sounds, and fluids. Will you be able to stomach it? Are you going to run away, faint, or do something else embarrassing?

Such fears are completely normal, and no surprise given this is probably your first viewing of a live-and-in-person birth. In the power of the moment, as you're helping your partner through her contractions, your anxieties may fade into the background. And when the baby crowns, you'll likely be too awestruck to notice the surrounding mess or commotion, completely forgetting to faint. Even if you do faint or throw up, you haven't failed anyone. There are plenty of medical personnel who will get you quickly back on your feet and back in the thick of things.

 Say, Dad

The sight of a baby—no, a person—emerging from my wife is the most incredible thing I have ever seen, and I feel privileged to have seen it. When my first son was born, my wife said that it was looking at my face as our son came out that motivated her to keep going. She says I looked so excited and amazed that it spurred her on. Far from being sidelined, this made me feel like I played a role (however small) in the birth.

—Simon Carswell, father

You'll have other intense reactions, too. You might feel afraid or angry when seeing the doctor wrestling your baby's shoulders out of the birth canal. This might be your first experience of being afraid for and protective of your child. While hard to feel, this is a great and worthwhile instinct. Still, trust the doctor will do what's right for your baby.

And if your partner has a caesarian section, you'll be worried about not only the baby but your partner as well. In most situations, the medical team invites the father to scrub up, enter the operating room, and observe the birth. However, that means you'll have to observe a doctor cut open your partner's abdomen. Once again, the experience of seeing your flesh and blood enter the world may trump any queasiness over seeing your partner's flesh and blood exposed—or it may not. If you're wondering whether to view a caesarian, be sure to talk it through with the doctor during the pregnancy office visits. Also, make a point of talking to some other dads who've been through a caesarian with their partners to get their perspectives and suggestions.

Whether it's a regular birth or a caesarian, being in the room or staying out are both legitimate and understandable decisions.

Taking an Active Role in the Delivery

Depending on where you deliver and how your doctor practices, you might be able to take a more active role during the birth itself if you want. For instance, some facilities and practitioners encourage, or at least allow, the dad to deliver the baby himself. The medical professionals remain in the room to coach you through delivery and provide quick backup if there are any problems. Fathers who've delivered their own babies describe it as profound, spiritual, indescribable, breathtaking, deeply moving, euphoric, or all of the above.

If you and your partner decide you want to do this, prepare ahead of time with your doctor. Don't forget to discuss the fact that you can't hold your partner's hand and look lovingly into her eyes if you're positioned down between her legs.

Even if you decide not to deliver the baby yourself, you and you partner should also discuss (ahead of time) where you'll stand at the moment of birth. Do you remain at her side to coach and comfort her, waiting until the doctor places the baby on your partner's chest to see him? Or do you leave your partner's side and position yourself over the doctor's shoulder to witness (and perhaps record on camera) the crowning and delivery?

Speaking of recording, give some thought to whether and how taking photos and video might interfere with the magnificent moments of your baby's birth. Your memory is a remarkable recorder of big life moments, especially when you experience them without distraction. No matter how many other children you have, this one is born exactly once. Cameras may help or hinder the experience—just be sure to immerse yourself fully into your baby's birth.

Say, Dad

Watching your husband become a father is really sexy and wonderful.

—Cindy Crawford

There may be situations when the doctor wants you to remain at your partner's side, usually with good reason. Your primary job is coaching and supporting your partner through delivery, even if you have the freedom to step away.

You're unlikely to step away once the baby arrives. Go ahead and touch him, hold him, talk to him, and otherwise welcome him into your life and family. Remember, your connection with this unique child starts right now and lasts a lifetime!

Push, Crown, Plop

The doctor will tell your partner when she should start pushing the baby out. Stay in the flow with her and the doctor. Help your partner reposition her body, if that's what the doctor needs. Ideally, you and the other team members are in synch with each other by now, working smoothly together. If you've never seen a delivery before, the midwife or doctor is there to guide you through. Ask questions and get reassurance as you go along.

College and pro coaches usually get more wound up as the game goes along: pacing, jumping, and screaming at the refs. Don't follow their example during labor and delivery! Stretch, move around, and keep your body loose. Frequently take a deep breath, say "AAAAAHhhhhh," and think positive thoughts, like: "Our baby is almost here!" You can even practice focused breathing like you did with your partner in childbirth classes. One important point of the focused breathing (like Lamaze) is relaxation. You may think relaxation and concentration are incompatible, but they're not. Relaxation during labor actually increases your concentration while conserving the physical, emotional, and mental energy you need.

If your partner's delivery goes the way everyone hopes, the baby's heaviest body part—the head—comes down the birth canal first. Nature is putting gravity to work for her.

Of course, it takes more than gravity to get the baby's head through that narrow opening. That's why the contractions keep coming and your partner has to push. It's also why the baby's skull is flexible, and often, he will move his head to get out more easily. This is why his head may seem misshapen—and his face may look like a little old man's—when he arrives.

 Baby Steps

Fortunately, your baby's skull remains soft after birth, so it eventually adapts and grows into a "normal" shape. As the baby's face fills out, he'll look less like old Benjamin Button, too.

As your partner keeps pushing, the doctor delivering the baby prepares to help the head out. They may have to adjust baby's position or use tools to facilitate this, or the baby may make his way out with little or no "outside" assistance. Usually, the doctor helps maneuver the shoulders through the opening. After that, the baby's narrower body parts have an easy glide down the chute.

If the birth emotionally overwhelms you or makes you physically dizzy, that's okay. Sit down for a moment. If you need a nurse or doctor's help, ask. They're used to this and know how to help you out.

Presenting Problems

Nature designed a woman's body and fetal development so that the baby is positioned head down (in other words, head first) for labor and delivery. Doctors call this a *normal presentation* (because the head will "present" itself first during the birth), and it's the least difficult delivery setup. However, actual childbirth doesn't always follow nature's design.

In what doctors call a *breech birth,* some other part of the baby's body tries to lead the way down the birth canal. There are a few types of breeching positions:

- *Traverse breech,* when the baby is situated sideways in the uterus, with his back toward the birth canal. The baby can't progress down to the cervix from this position.

- *Frank breech,* when the baby is bent at the waist, so that his feet are near his head and his butt is "presenting" up against the cervix.

- *Complete breech,* when the buttocks also face downward, but the baby's knees are bent so the feet are near the buttocks.

- *Incomplete* or *footling breech,* when the baby has a foot leading the way in the birth canal.

When dealing with a breech birth, the doctor can try to manipulate the baby into a better position by reaching up the birth canal or by maneuvering the mother's body. If that doesn't work, your partner probably will be on her way to the operating room for a caesarian.

Two other "presenting" problems can also lead to a caesarian. If the placenta blocks the exit from the uterus to the birth canal, that's called *placenta previa.* The baby can't find a detour of his own, so surgery is his way out.

Finally, a tangled (or "prolapsed") umbilical cord can wrap around the baby, limiting his ability to breathe at birth. The umbilical can also become crimped, threatening his lifeline during labor. The doctor may be able to free the cord with manual manipulation, but if not, emergency surgery will be ordered.

We're Not Done Yet

If you recall from Chapter 10, labor has three stages. Wait a minute, it only took two stages to get the baby. Did somebody pull a fast one?

No. Your partner's uterus isn't empty once the baby comes out. She still has to "deliver" the placenta (a.k.a. stage 3). Meanwhile, your baby will disconnect from the placenta, now that he's starting to breathe and feed on his own.

Cutting the Cord

Sometime during your partner's pregnancy, at least one person will ask you, "Are you gonna cut the cord?" They mean the umbilical cord, which connects the baby to the placenta before and immediately after his birth. It's almost always cut before a mom pushes the placenta itself out of her uterus.

Why would you want to cut the cord? It can be a powerful rite of passage into fatherhood and a concrete metaphor or symbol for introducing the child to the larger world—helping him learn that he can survive, thrive, and be at home here with your help. It is an intimate, symbolic, and amazing way to start that process and demonstrate your lifelong commitment to your child.

The procedure itself is fairly simple. Someone (usually a medical professional) clamps two spots on the cord, a few inches away from the baby's belly. You cut through in between the clamps; cutting there prevents excess bleeding. A stump remains attached to what will eventually become your child's belly button.

The umbilical cord has to be tough and resilient to work, so it may feel hard to cut—especially when you're acutely aware that this thing is still attached to your infant. Go ahead with confidence, knowing that the doctor is right there.

If you've never done anything like it before and are afraid something might go wrong, rest assured that cutting the umbilical cord doesn't hurt the baby. He's started breathing on his own and will soon use his own mouth to eat. Therefore, he no longer needs any connection to the placenta for oxygen or other nourishment.

You can't reach over the sterile field of surgery during a caesarean operation, which greatly reduces the chances you can cut the cord. Talk it over ahead of time with the doctor, to see if there is any possibility you can do the honors. If so, make sure your desires are clear on the birth plan (see Chapter 10).

If you choose not to cut the cord, that's fine, too. You don't have to justify your decision to anyone else. You will still bond with your baby, and his birth itself is still a powerful rite of passage into fatherhood.

The Last Stage

Hormones are still working to maintain your partner's contractions so she'll "deliver" the placenta. Finished keeping the fetus alive, the placenta detaches from the uterine wall after birth.

After assuring the baby is fine, the doctor will shift to getting the placenta. You may need to divert your attention from the baby for a few minutes to coach your partner through delivering the placenta.

The placenta is worth looking at, even if it seems a bit gross to you. Only during pregnancy and childbirth does the human body create an organ (the placenta) and then get rid of that organ on its own. Isn't female anatomy amazing?

Some cultures have spiritual traditions or rituals for honoring the placenta—for example, burying it under a tree which the parents dedicate for the baby. This is a way of expressing gratitude for how the placenta sustained the child in the womb. If you and your partner are considering a placenta ritual, talk it over before delivery with your doctor, and check to see if any local ordinances limit what you can do.

Episiotomies and Other Fun

Because your baby had such a tight squeeze coming out the birth canal, the doctor might decide to widen the opening with an episiotomy. After injecting a numbing drug, the doctor makes a small cut in the tissue below your partner's vulva, known as the perineum. Once the placenta is delivered, the doctor sews up the incision.

The episiotomy used to be common practice, but fewer doctors perform them now. Some newer research suggests that mothers are better off without the incision and the pain of healing, even if they have minor perineum tears. Skipping the episiotomy doesn't seem to affect baby's health, and your partner has fewer infections.

On the other hand, a big tear in the perineum can be more painful than an episiotomy and take longer to heal. Recent data shows that a diagonal (or mediolateral) episiotomy may reduce the risk of the worst tears in the perineum. An episiotomy is necessary if the baby's shoulders don't deliver right after the head (a condition known as shoulder dystocia).

Ideally, the perineum has less healing to do without an incision. A smooth recovery may also mean your partner has less intercourse-related pain after pregnancy. That means your partner doesn't have to wait as long before having sex after childbirth—which may matter to you both!

During the pregnancy, find out where your doctor stands on doing an episiotomy, remembering that everyone's first priority is getting the baby out safely.

Emergency Delivery, Dad Style

To judge by movies and TV, babies are born in barns and backseats more often than in the hospital. Spoiler alert: that's not reality. Still, there's a slight chance you could end up in a situation that requires you to deliver your partner's baby on your own or without a doctor or nurse on the premises. Fortunately, you won't be alone—your partner is there, too.

Obviously, an emergency delivery isn't ideal. However, it may be safer than taking a dangerous car trip through floods, hurricanes, or blizzards to reach the hospital.

If it looks like you can't make it to a hospital or doctor quickly enough, call 911. The women and men who staff those phone lines are incredible and can tell you what to look for so you know if you need to deliver your child yourself. If that's the situation, they're also trained to walk you step by step through an emergency delivery. Simultaneously, they can get police and ambulance crews (also trained in birthing babies) headed to you ASAP. If you have time, you can also try to call your doctor. Keep in mind, however, that it's easier and safer in an emergency to follow one voice of guidance than it is to follow two or more.

Here are some signs it's time to step in:

- The baby's head is starting to crown

- Any other part of the baby's body or umbilical cord is visible

- Your partner absolutely can't keep herself from pushing, no matter how hard you both work to delay it

If you see any of those signs, situate your partner as comfortably as possible on a mattress, bed, or other soft surface. Whether in your house or in a vehicle, keep the heat up and use a spot that's as clean and accessible as you can find. Also, gather up blankets, coats, clothing, and any other coverings to keep her and the newborn warm. Don't worry about these items being "ruined." Delivering a baby is not as spotless as it appears on TV sitcoms—and not as grotesquely messy as a horror movie makes it. The bottom line is simple: the well-being of your baby and his mother are exponentially more vital than getting stains on the stuff you use to help you get the job done.

 Attention, Please

If the 911 dispatcher or doctor is coaching you through an emergency delivery, put your phone on speaker; that way, your hands are free and your partner can hear the instructions, too. Above all, don't hang up!

Helping Your Partner Through the Delivery

You may have difficulty imagining this, but you can (and must) remain calm during the delivery. As much as (or more than) your words, your calm and confidence tell your partner she can trust you and make it through. So keep communicating what's happening and what you're doing.

The goal is for her pushes to get your baby's head out and into your hands—that way, you can support the head while your partner pushes out the rest of the baby's body. You can then gently guide baby's shoulders out. But don't twist or pull on him; instead, let your partner's pushing provide the force.

As your baby comes out, you might see that the umbilical cord is wrapped around his head. Treat it (and the baby) gently, calmly passing the cord over his head. Never pull on or cut the cord while the baby is still in the birth canal.

Most emergency "amateur-delivery" childbirths have few complications. However, if you have questions or something doesn't seem right, tell 911 and follow the dispatcher's guidance.

 Attention, Please

There's an outside chance you'll need to perform CPR on the baby. Some childbirth classes teach infant CPR; you can also learn it from many hospitals and Red Cross chapters. This is a special skill you should have not only for an emergency home birth, but for any point during your child's infancy.

What to Do After Your Baby Arrives

Contrary to what you learned from old movies, don't hold the baby upside down or slap him. Instead, hold the baby with the head slightly lower than the feet to drain fluid from the nose and throat. You should see color in his skin as he starts breathing. If he doesn't begin to breathe, place the baby on his back and gently rub the chest or tap the bottoms of the feet. If that doesn't work, place your mouth over his nose *and* mouth and breathe repeatedly into his lungs to start resuscitation.

Once the baby is out, warm him up by gently rubbing him dry in soft towels or blankets. This helps your baby retain body heat and dries away the fluids that lubricated his way out. Your rubbing motions also help him begin to breathe regularly and make his blood flow.

Get the baby to your partner's breast as soon as you can, even before dealing with the umbilical cord. The body heat of your partner, coupled with sucking at her breasts, helps the baby stay warm and calm. Breastfeeding also triggers hormones that prompt your partner to deliver the placenta—and tell the uterus to contract, which reduces bleeding in there.

Once the baby is taken care of, you should then coach your partner through the delivery of the placenta. If possible, after your partner delivers it, save the placenta for examination at the hospital. You can place it in a plastic shopping bag or whatever else is handy.

You can now turn your attention back to the umbilical cord. The umbilical cord can stay attached if it looks like emergency personnel will get you to a hospital soon. However, if you won't be under a doctor's care for another hour or two, you should cut it.

To cut the umbilical cord, you'll do what the doctor would do in the hospital, only without the fancy clamps and knives:

- Wait until the cord stops pulsating; that will be your signal that it's no longer transporting blood from the placenta.

- Get two pieces of clean, thick string or shoelace, along with a sharp knife or a strong pair of scissors.

- Sterilize the knife and scissors for a few minutes in boiling water (see, you do need boiling water, just like in the movies!).

- Tightly tie one string around the cord about 4 inches from baby's belly, and the other string about 6 inches from the belly—leaving a 2-inch area for your cut.

- In the space between the two strings, cut the cord with your knife or scissors. Leave the cord stub on the baby as it is.

While you're doing all this, the police or EMTs should be on their way. Until they arrive, keep everyone as comfortable and warm as you can. Tell your partner she deserves a medal for heroism, hug the baby, and pat yourself on the back. If you melt down a little later, who can blame you?

While emergency daddy delivery is a last resort, remember that dads have helped moms birth babies for a long time. So the odds are good you can handle it if you have to.

The Least You Need to Know

- You're a key part of labor and delivery; you can act as an advocate for your partner and provide her with information from the doctor.
- Be smart and thoughtful about when and how you communicate news about your baby's birth.
- Use your birth plan, and simultaneously be ready to adapt to circumstances that arise.
- Stay fully involved in the birth by helping to deliver the baby or cutting the cord, even during a caesarean.
- If there's no other option, you can deliver your baby; nature (and 911) will guide you.

CHAPTER 12

Bringing Your Baby Home

In This Chapter

- Learning to trust your instincts
- Holding, changing, and soothing your baby
- Sharing the feeding duties with your partner
- Helping your partner adjust
- Showing off your baby

There's an infant in the car seat—in *your* car. Is this a dream? Is this a nightmare? Is this permanent?

Thoughts like this are normal. However, it's important to believe that what you see and feel today won't last forever. That requires a healthy dose of faith in the process of human development. Some days, you'll struggle to have this perspective. That's okay. At the same time, remember that you have (or can get) what you need to be a good father, no matter what happens next.

In this chapter, I give you some care tips for your baby, from changing a diaper to soothing her. I also discuss the emotional impact having a baby at home can have on you and your partner.

Nature Provides

Every day will fill to overflowing as you learn about your baby, practice taking care of her, and endlessly stare at her and her antics. You may not always see how fast she's changing, but after three or four weeks, look at photos from the day she was born. You'll see big differences.

Luckily, most babies also stay healthy during their first weeks, as if their bodies are too busy growing to have time for being sick. A baby who gains weight and wets her diaper every few hours is probably getting enough to eat. Breastfed babies tend to eat more often than bottle-fed ones, but the difference isn't always huge. She may develop an eating and sleeping schedule, but don't count on any such routine to last very long now, or over the next year.

Believe it or not, you (and your baby) can survive all this rapid change. The human species spent millennia producing parents and newborns. As a result, a lot of knowledge is built into your DNA and your instincts. For instance, when you bring your newborn home, your antennae are hypersensitive to anything the baby does or doesn't do. That's one way nature helps you meet the needs of this completely dependent little person.

Father instinct is real, powerful, and very useful. Most of the time, it's not that different from what you think of as mother instinct. In fact, French and British researchers recently demonstrated that fathers can recognize whether a crying baby is their own child just as reliably as mothers can. The key factor is how much time the parent spends with the child—not the parent's gender.

 Say, Dad

Becoming a father, I think it inevitably changes your perspective of life. I don't get nearly enough sleep. And the simplest things in life are completely satisfying.

—Hugh Jackman, actor

If you don't feel a sudden rush of father instinct, don't worry. Not all women get instant mother instinct, either. Time, experience, and the support of other parents will help you develop your fathering skills. Nature does provide!

Relax and Roll

The first few months demand a lot of time and attention for your baby. Nevertheless, make some time to take care of yourself. Nap when she's napping, and don't try to accomplish other major projects during your first few months of parenting.

Stay as open and relaxed as you can as you do things for and with the baby. For example, when caring for the baby, take every chance you can to feed, diaper, play with, burp, and put your infant down to sleep. This allows you to develop your own methods of comforting and coping with your child. Don't let your partner or other people "rescue" you too often, as she'll benefit greatly from having both your way and your partner's way work. You can avoid any interference by making sure you and your partner are aware of—and talk openly about—gatekeeping (more on this in Chapter 13).

Parenting requires a wide range of skills over time, and not every parent has a flair for every skill every day. For example, my wife found the first year with our babies maddening, because she had such a hard time figuring out what they wanted. "If only they would talk to me!" she would say. On the other hand, I discovered a previously unknown talent for (most of the time) sensing what the babies needed and then providing it. Their lack of language wasn't much of a barrier for me. However, when the girls got older, there were years when interactions came more easily to my wife than they did to me.

The point is this: neither you nor your partner has to do *everything* well. That's the benefit of "tag-teaming" with your partner—each of you can run with the things you do best while encouraging (and learning from) the things your partner does best.

While we're talking about learning .... as the author of a parenting advice book, I urge you to recognize that resources for parents of newborns are valuable when used in moderation. Sometimes, guidance from books, magazines, and websites will seem contradictory. The same thing goes for advice from friends and relatives. It may take practice, but learn to trust the instincts nature gives you. Combine your sense of what the baby needs with your overall common sense to sift through fathering and parenting advice.

Welcome information, and be willing to adopt new perspectives. However, don't treat everything you hear as gospel truth. If you do need help, though, you can call on your pediatrician, OB/GYN, and trustworthy friends and family members for help.

Daddy Sings the Blues

During the first few weeks, it's completely natural to feel out of sorts, blue, or even resentful of the demands your baby is making upon you. No matter how you feel over the first weeks and months of fatherhood, remember to take care of yourself, so you can for the baby and each other:

- Eat healthy to keep up your energy, focus, and mood. Make sure your partner eats well, too. If she's breastfeeding, she's still eating for two.

- Get exercise. Make sure you and your partner each have some time to get out of the house for a walk, run, or visit to the gym. Make time to exercise together, too—understanding that you won't be able to do it regularly for a while.

- Respect the fact that you or your partner may develop depression. The blues are normal, but if they linger, talk to your doctor and get help.

 Say, Dad

I went on a diet, swore off drinking and heavy eating, and in fourteen days I had lost exactly two weeks.

—Joe E. Lewis, comedian

A bout of the postbirth blues or struggling with the enormity of your new responsibilities may lead to resentment of the baby. This is an understandable response to the stress. However, remember that an infant cannot "decide" to make your life miserable. She's only responding to her most essential needs with instinct, not freely willed intention. So don't blame her for the stress.

Acknowledge how much work this is, and how much your life has changed. Get support to keep your perspective, so you don't let resentment cut you off from the joy that these days also include.

If you feel unusually depressed or unhappy, talk to your doctor. Postpartum depression can happen to mothers and fathers (more on this later in the chapter). If you feel so resentful of your baby that you're tempted to hurt her, contact your physician or a parenting "hotline" immediately. In addition, have a list ready of people who can come to give you an emergency break.

It's Hard to Break a Baby

My twin daughters were born prematurely and spent about a month in the neonatal intensive care unit. The NICU had nonstop activity and a lot of light. However, since we'd never had a baby before, we didn't realize that a NICU environment didn't provide a natural life rhythm for newborns.

So when one of our daughters slept 12 straight hours on her first day at home, and then three hours at a time for the next month, we were confused. Like any new parents, we looked in on our sleeping infants frequently to see if they were still breathing—sometimes waking them up in the process. This violated our pediatrician's first rule of parenting: Never wake a sleeping baby!

My point? Your instincts may seem like they're driving you to completely irrational behavior. Maybe so! Nevertheless, your instincts and early parenting experiences help you learn how resilient you—and your baby—can be.

Remember how the baby's skull is soft when she's born? Think of that as a symbol of how nature designs newborns to be flexible and hard to break. Infants need flexibility because they grow more rapidly now than at any other time of life.

This first year is a steady arc of growth in the baby's size, strength, and cognitive ability. Keep that in mind as you go through the sometimes confusing starts and stops of everyday baby care.

Holding Your Baby

You want to feed, burp, change, and do other things with the baby. Well, first you must learn how to pick her up, hold her, and set her back down. If no one taught you this skill as a kid and you didn't pick it up anywhere else, here are a few pointers.

 Say, Dad

There's no harm in a child crying; the harm is done only if his cries aren't answered. If you ignore a baby's signal for help, you don't teach him independence. What you teach him is that no other human being will take care of his needs.

—Dr. Lee Salk, child psychologist and author

Relax, especially the first few times you try it. Deep inside your DNA, the muscle memory of your forefathers will show the way! I have proof.

Recently, my infant grandson Sam and I visited some 30-something adults. I asked one young man if he'd like to hold Sam. He replied that he'd never held a baby before in his life, but he was willing to try.

He sat Sam on his lap and gingerly held his sides. Within a minute, the man's grip was more confident, and he was gently swaying Sam back and forth. Chuckling, he asked, "Why am I rocking the baby?" A couple of his friends laughed and said, "Human nature!"

Instinctively, at a level below his consciousness, this young man knew that rocking would keep Sam calm and happy. One of his female friends added, "If you hold Sam close to you, I bet instinct will guide you to hold his head against the left side of your chest—so he hears your heartbeat." Even without any experience, instinct kicked in and gave this man a way to help a baby he'd never met.

You, too, can master infant care if you relax enough to confidently combine your natural instinct with the baby's flexibility (and her naturally deep dependence on you).

Getting a Grip

If you aren't sure where to begin, here's a nitty-gritty guide to holding a baby who's currently lying down. (These instructions are for right-handed dads; just switch the descriptions if you're left-handed):

1. Put your right hand under the baby's neck, with your fingers opened wide. This will help you support her head and keep it from flopping around.

2. Put your left hand under the baby's bottom; don't be afraid to roll her body a little to get a firm hold.

3. Lift the baby with both hands, keeping the head slightly higher than the feet.

You may be nervous during the first few transfers from pick-up to a "hold" position, but you'll master this quickly if you stay calm and confident.

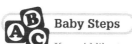 **Baby Steps**

If you'd like to see another example of how to hold a newborn, watch a fellow father demonstrate it in a short and very effective video at youtu.be/sVS-VvLMxvo.

Congratulations, you have successfully elevated your child! However, you will tire quickly if you continue to hold her at arm's length. Try shifting into one of these more comfortable positions:

The squirmy football: Place your baby's head in the crook of one elbow, and use that hand to support her butt. If her legs dangle down, no problem. Then, bend your arm and hold the baby close to your body like a football. Resist the urge to leap over furniture or crash into your brother as if he is a linebacker—at least while you're still holding the baby.

The cuddle: Keep your hands in the "pick-up" position with the baby facing you. Now, bring the baby toward you and hold her close to your chest, gently turning her head so she can breathe. This position can give you the unbeatable sensation of feeling your baby melt into you (and your heart) as she falls asleep. To comfort her, hum, purr, shush, or growl as you exhale; those vibrations in your chest remind your baby of being in the womb.

The bragger: Turn the baby around so she's facing outward. Use your right hand as a seat for your baby's butt while letting her legs dangle. Put your left hand firmly on her chest, so you're holding her torso and the back of her head close to your chest. Begin strutting around the neighborhood, proudly displaying your handiwork while (incidentally) letting your baby absorb the sights and sounds.

At some point, you'll need to lay the baby back down again. To do this, simply reverse whichever pick-up move you chose. Once the baby is on her back again, gently remove your hands from under her head and butt. Don't worry about the minor jostling involved; remember, she's flexible and resilient.

You're Both All Wet

By the time you're confident with your holds, the baby will need a bath. This is excellent timing, because holding a wet and soapy infant takes a lot of concentration.

Start by getting the baby tub and all of your supplies in place before you start running the water; you can't risk leaving the baby in the bath to retrieve something you need.

Pregnant Pause

Never leave the baby during a bath, and make sure she is secure within the tub. That may take two sets of hands when she's tiny.

If neither of you have bathed an infant before, invite an experienced parent to coach you the first time or two. If you don't mind taking instruction from your mother, bring her over.

Do *not* expect baby baths to be tidy. You and the surroundings will be damp when you're done. This is normal, so roll with it.

An infant's skin is very sensitive, so use mild soaps along with very soft towels and washcloths. Since the baby isn't yet climbing trees or rolling around in the dirt, you don't have to scrub her clean.

Eventually, the baby will learn to sit up, meaning she'll be less likely to flop and slide around during a bath. However, she will be more likely to squirm. Usually, frequent baths help the baby get used to and enjoy the water.

Lay out a clean, dry, soft towel on the floor, and lay the baby on it as soon as she comes out of the bath. Wrap the towel around her and then snuggle her close to prevent the chills. Infants usually love this part of the process, and it's fun for you, too.

Changing a Diaper and Watching Out for Diaper Rash

In early fatherhood, you'll change many things—including diapers. With luck, you'll also change the aversion you might currently have toward the sight, smell, and texture of human excrement (a.k.a. poop).

Like adults, babies pee more often than they poop. Over the first few months, there may be little or no odor from either, especially if your baby is breastfeeding. While stink free early on, your baby's poop will look alien—greenish and somewhere between liquid and smooth. Before long (and especially once the baby starts on solid food), poop gets brown and less fluid, although not solid.

Your baby gets her first diaper from a professional in the hospital. From then on, it's up to you, and nearly every diaper you open will contain something it didn't have when it went on the baby.

In theory, you've already arranged a changing table with clean diapers, ointment, wipes, and a disposal container within easy reach.

Now it's time to lay your baby on the changing table and use these supplies.

Are you ready to make a mess? Have you practiced holding your breath? Let's begin:

First, open the diaper, pulling the front half downward and through your baby's legs. Gently grasp the baby's ankles and pull her legs and butt up off the table, just high enough to get the entire diaper out from under her. Put the wet or dirty diaper out of baby's reach. You don't have to deal with that one now—your baby needs your attention first.

 Baby Steps

Changing a diaper gives you excellent face time with your baby. Entertain and distract her with chatter, songs, noises, funny faces, kisses, and whatever else you can think of.

Next, use a washcloth or baby wipes to clean off all the skin on and around the baby's bottom, anus, vagina or scrotum, legs, back, and all the cracks and folds covered up by the diaper. Clean every spot every time; otherwise, diaper rash will quickly appear. Diaper rash will happen anyway, but thorough cleaning can reduce its frequency. Dry all the skin before you put on ointment or a new diaper. Moisture—especially on skin where you apply ointment—accelerates diaper rash.

After that, grab a clean, dry diaper. Gently grab her ankles again, and lift her butt in the air so you can position the new diaper with your other hand. Adjust your baby and the diaper so her waist and the top of the diaper align with each other. Then, settle the baby down in place.

Fortunately, infants don't squirm much on the changing table during the first few weeks. That gives you time to learn diaper basics before the looming days when you must wrangle your baby and her diapers during every change.

Finally, pull the diaper front up through the baby's legs, using the snaps or Velcro to get a snug fit. Don't make it uncomfortably tight (she'll be unhappy) or too lose (you'll be unhappy when the diaper leaks onto the baby's clothes and you).

Once you've got the baby dressed and in the crib, your partner's arms, or another safe place, you can deal with the dirty or wet diaper. You should also clean off the changing table so you don't have to battle this diaper's mess when you return to change the next one. If the baby wipes aren't flushable, dump them (and disposable diapers) in a plastic bag you can seal up later before putting it in the trash. Diaper and wipe odors annoy the neighbors unless they are well contained (the diapers, not the neighbors).

A wet cloth diaper can go straight into the dirty diaper can or bag. A poopy cloth diaper needs rinsing first. The simplest method: swish it around in the toilet bowl until most of the poop breaks free. If you flush while rinsing, hold on tight to the diaper itself—let go, and the resulting clog will disable the toilet and dictate a visit from the plumber.

Once you change a few diapers, you'll realize that these instructions take longer to read than they do to carry out. Changing will be second nature in no time.

Now that I've walked you through how to change your baby's diaper, let me tell you more about diaper rash. Diaper rash generates a shade of red—and discomfort—you won't find anywhere else in nature. When moisture is held against the skin (for example, by a diaper), bacteria forms. These bacteria generate ammonia that irritates a baby's sensitive skin and creates diaper rash. Antibiotics are also known to cause diaper rash.

 Pregnant Pause

Disposable diapers tend to generate more diaper rash than cloth ones, because the plastic in disposables can make your baby sweat more, adding to the crotch moisture. Cloth diapers can also irritate your baby's skin and cause diaper rash if they aren't soft and free of fragrances.

As I mentioned earlier, there are ways you can help protect your baby against diaper rash. Change diapers regularly—you'll get the rhythm with experience—cleaning and drying baby's bottom and crotch completely each time. In addition, consider extending "naked baby" time, so your baby's skin can air out. For naked baby boys, lay a washcloth over his penis to contain spontaneous spurts of pee. And if you use cloth diapers, wash them in gentle, dye-free, and fragrance-free detergent and very hot water.

When a rash does develop, treat it promptly and aggressively. Cover the sore spots with diaper ointment. Make sure the skin is dry first; otherwise, the ointment traps the moisture, which makes things worse. You may be tempted to use baby powder or talc to dry the baby's skin. However, doctors frown on this—the powder can be inhaled and create breathing problems for your baby. If your doctor prescribes an antibiotic for baby and it causes diaper rash, keep treating the rash with ointment. However, don't discontinue the antibiotic if your baby needs it.

Cleaning the Cord Stump

Most umbilical cords dry up and fall off within baby's first few weeks, leaving behind a small stump. Until it falls off, clean the cord stump with mild soap and water. You shouldn't submerge it in water, so give your baby sponge baths during the first few weeks. After it's clean, dry it thoroughly. Some doctors suggest using a cotton swab dipped in alcohol to wipe the base gently in order to help prevent infection. However, the use of alcohol around the umbilical stump is not a universal practice. Parents should follow their pediatrician's recommendation on this.

You may also need to alter how often you diaper your baby so you can keep it as clean and dry as possible.

Some drainage or bleeding are normal, but if you have questions or worry that something isn't right with the area, talk to your doctor.

Soothing Your Baby

News flash: babies get upset and cry. The five primary reasons they do this are the following:

1. They're hungry.

2. They're tired.

3. The diaper is soiled or wet.

4. They have gas or are sick.

5. Who the heck knows?

The first few weeks at home may feel a bit like torture as you try to distinguish your baby's hungry cry from her tired cry. Be patient; you will get the hang of it. Most of the time, you'll ease her distress by changing, feeding, or helping her fall asleep.

 Pregnant Pause

Invest in a good flashlight to have by your bed in case the power goes out. A friend once got up in the middle of the night to get his crying infant and broke his nose walking into the closed nursery door. Make sure you can see what you're doing, especially when you're tired.

However, there will be times when, after doing all those things, your infant is still upset. Neither you nor your partner will be able to figure out why, and worst of all, she won't be able to tell you. That's when you have to ride it out and comfort her as best you can for as long as you can—and then a little bit longer.

To get through these confusing and frustrating times, you should develop some soothing strategies. The following are some ideas for you to try; however, recognize that a trick which works tonight might not work in the morning:

ID the problem. Check the diaper, feed her, or try a pacifier. This is trial and error at first, but it also helps you start to tell the different cries apart from one another.

Embarrass yourself. Make funny noises and funny faces. Tap your memory and sing tunes from the campfire, The Clash, Perry Como, Chopin, Mariah Carey, Mary Chapin Carpenter—whatever works to distract and settle baby down. Randomly created nonsense songs work, too. For example, my daughter and son have a friend named Yasuhiro who brings his ukulele when babysitting my grandson, Sam. When trying to get Sam to take a bottle from me, I started singing a made-up song which went, "Yasu plays the ukulele, Yasu plays the ukulele. Sometimes he plucks and sometimes he strums. Someday soon, he'll learn to play the drums." Other grownups in the room laughed, but Sam started sucking! My Yasu tune worked for about a month before I needed to come up with some other silliness to "sing."

Hold your baby close and move around. Swing around, dance gently, bounce on a yoga ball, or rock in a rocking chair. Experiment with what you have around the house and what your instinct encourages you to try. If you'd like some tips, search online; for example, this video is one way to hold a fussy baby: youtube.com/watch?v=ofPeo-g06Ak.

Swaddle. Wrap your baby up in a specially designed swaddle or use a simple baby blanket (see Chapter 8 for more about swaddles and swaddling). Swaddling gives your baby security and warmth while also minimizing the normal "starts" that can disturb her sleep.

Go for a walk. Bundle your baby up in an infant carrier and take her for a stroll. The natural rhythm of your steps reminds her of being in the womb, which was a very comfy place.

Be your baby's pacifier. Some babies like to suck on a parent's finger, arm, shoulder, shirt, and so on. If you try this, just make sure your fingernails won't scratch the inside of her mouth—that's a surefire wail inducer.

Your soothing methods may or may not be different from the methods your partner or other relatives use—that's entirely fine. In fact, it's healthy for the baby to learn how to be comforted in multiple ways. That builds resiliency and gives her practice with different means she can use in a few months when it's time to comfort herself at bedtime.

Sleeping

Your newborn will sleep a lot of the time, but not for long stretches. The American Academy of Pediatrics puts it simply and succinctly: "An infant who wakes frequently is normal and should not be perceived as a poor sleeper." Your baby may only stay awake for an hour or so before napping again.

 Attention, Please

The National Institute of Child Health and Human Development says newborns sleep or drowse for 16 to 20 hours a day (day and night).

Not only is your infant's internal "clock" adjusting to life outside the womb, her tummy is still tiny, so hunger will wake her more often than when she's older and can take in more food. She's unlikely to sleep more than four hours before getting hungry, and research indicates that breastfed babies will wake up hungry a bit more often than formula-fed ones.

Go with her flow, remembering that your sleep clock will be fouled up for a while, too. She's not trying to make your life miserable; her body is responding to her needs for rest, just as it does for food.

When you put her down to sleep in the crib, make sure she's on her back. Some parents worry that the baby will be uncomfortable sleeping on her back, but the research shows that babies are less likely to stir or wake up than when sleeping on their stomachs. Plus, putting her on her back reduces the possibility of Sudden Infant Death Syndrome (SIDS). She may cough or appear to be gagging while sleeping, but in nearly all cases, she isn't going to choke. Healthy infants naturally swallow or cough up fluids, an example of the essential (and healthy) human gag reflex. The opening to the windpipe works in a way that makes it unlikely for fluids to cause choking. So she may actually clear congestion *better* when on her back.

As your baby gets older, she'll probably start sleeping for longer stretches. By then, it helps to develop sleep time routines. Start a while before bedtime to ramp down vigorous and loud activity. Consider singing, reading her a book, rocking, and so on. However, don't get rigidly hung up on routines during the first month or so, as it usually takes a few months before the baby will respond to more formal "sleep training" and learn how to lay calmly in her crib before and after a nap. Remember, the goal of sleep training is meeting your child's needs and having nighttime routines you can cope with. If your baby isn't sleeping through the night by 6 or 12 months, there's probably nothing wrong with her. Babies just develop skills at different rates!

If you have any questions or concerns about your baby's sleeping habits, your pediatrician and her staff should be willing to answer them. (If they aren't willing, find another physician.)

Feeding

As an involved dad, you'll be part of a parenting team that closely tracks what and when your baby is eating (actually, at this stage, she's just drinking).

Newborns need plenty of nourishment because they're burning through calories in order to grow, stay warm, and build enough strength to eat the next meal. Because your baby's stomach is small in size, it fills quickly—and needs regular refilling.

Your infant may eat every hour or two or have longer intervals between feedings. Those intervals will change, often without notice, depending on what she needs. It's usually wiser to watch for your baby's satisfaction level rather than the clock. And frequent feeding means frequent interruption of your sleep. Stay relaxed on the days your infant has to eat 10 times in 24 hours; getting annoyed won't change how hungry she is.

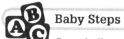 **Baby Steps**

One challenge for many new parents is getting their infant to suck successfully and consistently. Nurses, midwives, lactation consultants, and experienced parents can give you tips to help, even if your baby is bottle fed.

Some dads think that meals are the mom's problem (especially if she's breastfeeding), because it's her job to keep Junior full. Not so; you still have a vital role to play. Feeding your baby is a powerful way to connect and strengthen your special father-child bond. The more you are involved in the feeding routine, the more you strengthen the baby's association of "nourishment" with both you and your partner.

How can you possibly be a central player?

- Burp the baby while your partner feeds her.

- Your partner pumps her breast milk for a bottle. This allows you to feed—and teaches your baby to drink from a bottle. (Wait until your baby is latching well at the breast before trying this.)

- Take regular feeding shifts, delivering the meal through a bottle of breast milk or formula. This builds your intimacy with your baby and gives your partner a break.

Getting and staying involved may mean challenging attitudes and habits that are familiar to you, your partner, and many other people. However, feeding (even breastfeeding) isn't just for moms!

With practice and patience, you'll get good at feeding your baby. To feed your baby, sit on a comfortable piece with a solid arm on which you can support your nondominant (and nonfurniture) arm. Set your baby's neck and lower head in the crook of your nondominant elbow, using the lower arm and hand to hold her close to your body.

Use your dominant hand to guide the bottle into your baby's mouth. Babies have a natural sucking instinct, but it may take many repetitions before she gets the hang of sucking on this kind of nipple—just as it can take time for her to synch up with your partner's nipples. Do your best to stay calm; when you tense up, so does the baby, making it harder for her to suck.

To help your baby, you may have to rock her or get up and walk around to distract and comfort her while you slip the nipple in. Gently stroking her cheek with one of your spare fingers might also trigger sucking. Chat and sing if that seems to work.

Say, Dad

Being a role model is the most powerful form of educating … too often fathers neglect it because they get so caught up in making a living they forget to make a life.

—John Wooden, Hall of Fame basketball coach

Be prepared for long hauls in the beginning. It might take close to an hour to feed her 4 or 6 ounces at first, and there may be loud crying. Check for tension in your baby's body, and remember to stay as relaxed as you can, with your feet in a wide, strong stance.

On the other hand, your baby may take to bottle feeding with little or no trouble. It all depends on the kid.

Even if you do have agonizing days, don't take it personally. She's not telling you that you're inept. Instead, she's saying she doesn't know how to do this yet, and she needs Daddy to help her learn.

Stick to this routine, even if people question your judgment or say it's inappropriate for a dad to "horn in on" breastfeeding to feed his infant. Feel free to think of such folks as clueless.

Breast or Bottle?

Nearly all research supports the notion that breast milk is better overall for your baby than formula. That's not surprising, since it was the only method for the eons of human existence before Henri Nestlé invented manufactured formula in 1867.

The chemical composition of breast milk adapts to the newborn's needs, for example, by giving baby's immune system a boost during the first days of life. Breast milk is also easy on a newborn's developing digestive system. In most cases, a mother's milk supply miraculously corresponds to how hungry the baby is.

Nevertheless, breastfeeding will be new for both your baby and your partner. Your baby may suck successfully from day one or take a couple of weeks to "latch" consistently. If your partner and your baby have trouble getting in synch, the best things you can do are the following:

- Keep the atmosphere calm.

- Avoid criticizing or judging your partner's technique (even nonverbally).

- Take the baby for burping and comforting, so your partner has time to regroup and relax.

- Acknowledge, and express gratitude for, her perseverance.

- Encourage her to call on a lactation consultant, a visiting nurse, the pediatrician, or other resources for support and guidance. Join your partner in these meetings, so you can learn new ways to support her.

There's nothing wrong with your partner if breastfeeding doesn't succeed or if she has no interest in trying it in the first place. Don't pass judgment on her, and ignore anyone else who might.

Fortunately, your baby can also grow normally and in good health if you feed her formula. Consult with your pediatrician about which kind of formula will work best for your baby's needs. If you or the doctor discovers your baby has food allergies, you can purchase specialized formula, or even make your own.

Bottle Washer

Bottles take maintenance. Because your partner has fewer nipples and no containers to wash, breastfeeding has substantial conveniences. (She certainly won't be competing with pots and pans for space in the dish drainer.) However, your partner must be with the baby in order for breastfeeding to work—not always convenient, especially for her. So no matter what, you're going to have baby bottles in your life.

Be prepared to sacrifice substantial kitchen counter space to washing and drying all the components of bottles and breast pumps. Breast pumps come with plastic parts, including a conelike funnel that attaches to the breast, narrow hoses, holders onto which you thread a bottle, and other stuff. Bottles come with bottles (of course), lids, collars, and nipples. Many infant bottles have a two-piece nipple, with an inside "regulator" to slow the flow of milk.

Before using any of these plastic parts for the first time, follow the manufacturer's instructions for sterilization. That usually means putting the pieces in a pot of water. Make sure the water is deep enough to cover all the pieces, then boil them for 15 to 20 minutes.

Once you're using the equipment, take the lead in keeping all of it clean. After using a bottle or breast pump, wash each part separately. Yes, it can be a pain in the butt, but thorough cleaning cuts down on how often your baby gets sick.

Pregnant Pause

If your home uses well water, plan to sterilize your gear about once a month, since your regular washing routine won't eliminate mineral build-up.

Start by rinsing everything to clear out the milk and residue. Then fill the sink or any other clean container with hot water and add mild, scent-free dish soap. If you have time, let everything soak for a bit.

To scrub out bottles, many parents keep a "dedicated" sponge for use only with them. A bottle brush also makes it much easier to reach all parts of the bottle and clean it completely. You can even use a very small brush to clean inside the nipples; read the instructions for the nipples, however, to see if using that kind of brush might damage them.

You can put modern-day bottles and the accompanying parts in the top rack of a dishwasher, but you need some way to contain them.

Get a dishwasher basket to hold the smaller parts, as the lightweight nipples and lids are especially prone to flying all over inside the machine.

Whether you wash in the sink or the dishwasher, let the bottles and other parts air dry. Most stores with infant gear sell various contraptions you can use to stand or prop up all your parts as they dry.

Burping and What It Brings

During your baby's first few months, she will swallow air along with milk as she eats. That's normal; it takes a while for her to develop the muscle memory needed to get the food into her tummy while keeping the air out.

Ever had a bad case of gas that you just couldn't find a way to get rid of? It's uncomfortable and sometimes very painful. Your baby has a similar experience when there's air in her digestive system—hence the need for grown-ups to burp babies. Burping releases bubbles and air pockets, producing burps, along with partially digested milk that people affectionately call "spit-up." It's good policy to always have a cloth diaper nearby to catch the residue—or wipe up what you don't catch.

Say, Dad

When your baby is beautiful and perfect, never cries or fusses, sleeps on schedule and burps on demand, an angel all the time, then you're the grandma.

—Teresa Bloomingdale, mothering author

The normal routine calls for burping the baby about halfway through a feeding, and again when the feeding ends. In addition to relieving pain, the "halfway" burp frees up room for more food to satisfy your baby's hunger.

Despite what you've seen on TV and in the movies, vigorous whacks on the baby's back are ineffective, and they hurt. Successful burping techniques all use gentle touch, either through rubbing or patting. Experiment with one or more of these positions:

- Sit up straight and hold the baby on one side of your body, with her chin on your shoulder. Use your other hand to pat or rub her back. The motion of a rocker may help when sitting.

- Using the same over-the-shoulder technique as you do while sitting, stand up and walk around. Gentle bouncing and rocking motions can also help. Make sure you have a firm grip on your baby!

- Lay the baby across your lap, on her stomach. Holding her head higher than her chest, pat or rub on her back. If she spits up, watch your step.

- Sit the baby upright in your lap, cradling her chin in one hand. Use the other hand to rub or pat her back. Once again, moving the baby gently back and forth can help.

Getting your baby to burp can be very satisfying. If she's been fussy, she's liable to calm right down, relaxing in your warm and competent arms.

Mommy Care

You and your partner go through huge emotional and psychological adjustments once you become parents. Meanwhile, your partner's body is also recovering and healing from pregnancy and childbirth. Perhaps she's recovering from a C-section. On top of that, her hormones are still operating in ways that neither one of you is used to. With such a combination, she may worry she's letting you down or falling behind in caring for the baby.

So don't be surprised if you both feel extra stressed, and if she needs extra TLC from you and other people (like her own mother).

Telling Tired from Depressed

If you recall from earlier in the chapter, both moms and dads can have the "baby blues" from time to time after the baby arrives. However, your partner is usually more likely to struggle with this, thanks to hormones and the ordeal of childbirth.

She may have mood swings and feel sad, anxious, or overwhelmed. She might lose her appetite, have crying jags, or have trouble sleeping.

The difference between baby blues and postpartum depression is time and severity. If this is just baby blues, these symptoms often fade away within a few days or a week and there's no need for treatment. The symptoms of postpartum depression last longer and are more intense.

 Pregnant Pause

If you or your partner is battling depression, don't wait to ask for help. Depression is a biochemical problem, not a moral or spiritual failure. Like a broken leg, depression is treatable, so if you have it, get it treated.

Instead of simple sadness, your partner may also feel hopeless and worthless. Her interest in the baby may diminish or disappear. She may even think about or worry about hurting herself or the baby. And in extreme (and rare) instances, she can develop hallucinations or act on the urge to inflict harm. Those severe cases call for immediate intervention, and often a hospital stay.

But why would a woman get depressed after the miracle of having a baby?

- Dramatic change in hormone levels, just as minor hormone shifts impact her mood before menstruation

- Exhaustion from the delivery and lack of restful sleep

- Feeling overwhelmed by the responsibility of caring for the baby or feeling inadequate about it

- Stress over the changes in her career and sense of personal identity

- Feeling less attractive

- Having little, if any, free time

- Distorted or unrealistic expectations of what being a "good" mother means

None of these is the single, undeniable "cause" of postpartum depression, and no one has identified a surefire cause. However, to successfully support your partner, *why* she has postpartum depression is much less important than *how* you respond to it.

Start by recognizing you can't argue someone out of depression any more than you can debate someone out of diabetes. Depression is symptomatic of biochemical imbalances—in other words, it's a disease.

Postpartum depression can begin anytime within the first year after childbirth. And if your partner had depression before she got pregnant, she faces a higher risk for postpartum depression. If you think your partner has it, get help from your health-care provider. Antidepressants and other drug therapies can help, especially when combined with "talk" therapy under the care of a licensed counselor or psychologist.

We Time

By now, you know that caring for your newborn is all-consuming. (If you don't realize that yet, please start the book over!) Parenting will continue to dominate the lives of you and your partner for many years to come.

Does this leave any room for nourishing your relationship with each other? Yes, but only if you make the room. If you hope to maintain your romantic and co-parenting relationship, making time and space for each other is non-negotiable. In addition, you each need time for yourselves, friends, family, work, and other activities.

Perhaps the first thing to accept is this: there will be less time available for these important events than you had previously. Therefore, you have to manage this precious time more effectively and creatively than before.

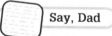

Say, Dad

Children aren't happy with nothing to ignore,
And that's what parents were created for.

—Ogden Nash, poet

Because there's more to your relationship than sex, your time together with your partner should not be exclusively for having sex. (However, it doesn't always have to exclude sex either!)

Think and act creatively and flexibly. For example, you and your partner can grab small bits of time together when the baby is asleep. Maybe it's a tranquil conversation about tomorrow's schedule, a raucous recounting of the baby's antics that afternoon, or a quiet few minutes of cuddling on the couch.

You can also take time to text or call each other a few times during the day. It feels good to get word that someone you love is thinking about you.

Once the baby is eating and sleeping with some predictability, recruit one (or more) of your parents, siblings, or friends to come over to watch the baby for an hour or two while you and your partner do one of the following:

- Take a nap.

- Go for a walk.

- Get a pizza and a beer.

- Wander around the mall.

- Visit the gym.

- Run errands.

- Grab coffee with a friend.

- Go to the movies.

Don't expect huge chunks of baby-free time during the first six months or so. For example, a second honeymoon in Maui might be unrealistic—unless you live in Lahaina, in which case you should consider a staycation. Just make sure you and your partner are able to get away for a little bit and enjoy each other's company.

The Traveling Baby Show

With the baby as a "star" on the family scene, she (and you) will be in great demand to bring her around for well-deserved oohs and ahhs. Especially in the early weeks, traveling with the baby may make you feel like you're in a poorly managed circus. Eventually, you will get the hang of preparing for trips (whether short or long) with sufficient food, diapers, clothes, and the like.

Stroller Safety

Wherever you go with the baby, you'll still have to transport her once you get there. You'll come to rely a lot on your stroller, so it's important to get the hang of folding, stowing, and unfolding the stroller on these outings. Always follow these simple safety steps when using a stroller:

- Secure the baby with shoulder and belt straps.

- Don't risk tipping the stroller over by hanging bags on the handles; use the storage area instead.

- Lock the wheels every time you stop.

- Keep your baby's fingers and toes away from "pinchable" spots when folding or unfolding the stroller.

- Double-check that the locking device is secure, so you avoid accidental fold-ups while in motion.

- Follow the manufacturer's instructions and recommendations. Really!

Once you arrive at your destination pushing your baby in the stroller, be prepared for family and friends to be as captivated with your baby as you are … or almost as captivated, anyway.

Airborne Babies

The odds are good that you or your partner lives far away from at least one of your parents, siblings, or close friends. All things being equal, it's easier for the distant (adult) relative to travel to your town to meet the baby. However, all things are not equal—one of your parents may be too unwell to travel; your brother may have three small kids of his own and be unable to afford the time, money, and hassle to bring them; or a loved one may be getting married 10 days after the baby came.

Therefore, in the first few weeks or months of your child's life, you may face the challenge of taking an infant on an airplane. This is usually stressful, especially the first time. However, there are good ways to prepare, including the following:

- Pack smart (more on that in a minute).

- Use social media to "borrow in advance" a car seat, stroller, crib, or other gear from someone who lives in/near where you're going. This saves you from having to haul as much on your journey.

- Ask the people you'll visit to lay in a supply of diapers, bottles, formula, pacifiers, and baby toys.

- Contact your airline ahead of time to ask how they can accommodate you for the flight.

- If at all possible, fly nonstop. It's best to only get on and off the plane once.

- Have a friend or relative take you to the airport and help you check the luggage.

- Make sure the driver who picks you up at the destination airport has the right kind and size of car seat already installed for your baby.

- Look for family-friendly resources in the airport itself, such as family bathrooms and dedicated security lines for families. If there's not a special line, ask a TSA agent to let you skip ahead in line.

- Avoid wearing a belt, shoes with shoelaces, a heavy jacket, or anything else you have to take off to pass through security (and put back on later). The same goes for your baby (sometimes, TSA really does make you remove an infant's shoes).

- Spread out in the waiting area. New parentage gives you social permission to use more than one chair, lay the baby on the floor, and the like.

 Attention, Please

The Transportation Security Agency (TSA) allows parents to carry on more than 3.4 ounces (100 ml) of "medically necessary" liquids and gels for a baby. This includes medications, baby formula, baby food, and breast milk. In addition, these items are not required to be in a zip-top bag.

Packing is key to a successful (or, at least, minimally stressful) trip. Believe it or not, you can pack light. You don't need to bring every last baby item, especially if folks on the other end are helping provide some—and there's a Target nearby them. Pack simple, easy-to-wash clothing for you, your partner, and the baby. Think ahead and keep it simple. For instance, if you're traveling because your partner is in a wedding, ship her fancy dress and shoes ahead of time, rather than taking them on the plane.

Also, remember that folks will be excited to meet your baby—and give her presents. So you'll probably come back home with more stuff than you left with.

You will have a handful of baby on the plane, so the less you have to carry (and keep track of), the better. Strive to have only one carry-on for the baby, with the following items:

- Several bottles, if your partner isn't breastfeeding

- Ready-to-drink formula, rather than the kind you'd need to mix at an airport water fountain, or in the miniscule airplane bathroom

- Any medications, infant Tylenol, or other items the baby needs

- Four pacifiers, in case one rolls under a seat or down the aisle

- Bibs and washcloths (the number depends on the length of your trip)

- A baby blanket, to keep her warm when she sleeps and provide privacy when nursing

- Toys or anything else that can distract her

- Any small item that can remind you and your partner to relax

When entering and exiting the aircraft, wear your infant. Carrying her in a snugglie or Moby helps keep her calm, while keeping your hands free to maneuver to your seats. You can also use it during the flight to walk the baby up and down the aisle or keep her warm, calm, and napping while you sit. Ask for help from flight attendants; most of them find babies to be fun, and know how to lend new parents a hand.

While changing a diaper, feeding, or making silly talk with your baby, be polite to others. However, don't be intimidated by (or confrontational with) other people who don't like the sight of dirty diapers or breastfeeding. It's not like they didn't poop in their diapers way back when!

Infant ears tend to be very sensitive to the changes in cabin pressure when the plane is taking off and landing. If you've ever had similar problems, you know the pain can be excruciating, even for an adult. Keep your infant sucking on a pacifier or bottle during take-off and landing, since this tends to release pressure in the inner ear. Some babies do fine if they are already asleep, but be prepared for a quick response, no matter what.

Setting Boundaries for Visits with Your Baby

Becoming parents gives you both new authority over where and how you spend time with other people. But first, you and your partner need to figure out what works well for your baby and you.

Let's say your parents want to drop in unannounced to visit the baby. Your partner feels jazzed about the idea because she loves your parents—they energize her, and she knows they'll take the baby off her hands for a spell. However, you find drop-in visits annoying because you feel they don't respect your time and personal space. Plus, you think all these grandparent visits are crowding your father-baby time.

If you and your partner both favor (or oppose) this kind of visit, your course is simplified. However, if one likes it and the other doesn't, which side you're on matters less than striking a compromise.

For example, in the scenario I described, you two could decide (together!) that Grandpa and Grandma can come as often as they like, but they have to call ahead—that way, you can tell them if the baby just went to sleep or if he's wide awake and eager to see them. Another option is to set a limit of two or three unannounced visits per week. You could also decide to defer entirely to your partner's desires—or vice versa.

The first step is to know what you want, realizing that your needs and desires may change next week or next month.

The second step is communicating your desires, needs, limits, and rules in clear, honest, and respectful words to each family member and friend likely to be affected. Don't pull your punches or beat around the bush. Be calm, straightforward, and realistic. Don't assume that your dad will pass the message on to Aunt Latoya without you needing to talk to her—or, rather, don't assume that Aunt Latoya will get exactly the message you intended for her to get.

The third and final step is sticking to your guns. Don't send mixed messages by relaxing your requirements too soon. Sure, you can adjust as time goes on, the baby gets older, and situations change. But in the beginning, make clear that you and your partner hold ultimate responsibility for the baby—and you want others to respect that fact.

Remember, showing off the baby is supposed to be fun!

The Least You Need to Know

- Your own instincts and intuition are valuable tools for you, your partner, and the baby.
- You can soothe, hold, feed, and change your baby as well as (or better) than anyone. Plus, the time spent with your baby bonds you two even more.
- Make sure to support your partner through the early days of parenting by finding some free time to spend with her and watching for signs of depression.
- Make your desires known about guests after the baby is born.

CHAPTER 13

Making Your Family

In This Chapter

- Developing strong, positive attitudes toward fatherhood
- Creating your fathering vision statement
- Considering attitudes on marriage and family
- Fencing out gatekeeping
- Raising a child with birth defects

During the pregnancy and delivery of your baby, you're participating in an amazing process, even during the times it's difficult. So what will happen once your baby is actually born?

Spoiler alert: You'll be participating in an amazing process, even during the times it's difficult.

In this chapter, I discuss ways you can stay open to the good stuff, get practical support for being an involved dad from your partner (and others), develop a vision for your own fathering, and take care of a child with special needs.

Your Fathering Approach

In your life as a father, there are many circumstances you can't control. Fortunately, "control" isn't necessary to be a good father—or to live a good life, for that matter. Instead, good and effective fathers nurture acceptance and contrasting responses to the people, places, and things of life.

Father Attitudes

Openness to the excitement and miracle of having a child to nurture requires some practice, even for the most enlightened among us. Tune up your amazement muscles early on, because there are even more miracles ahead in helping your newborn grow into the remarkable person he will be.

While getting used to this change in your life, you may have moments (or even days) when you're astounded by the following:

- You and your partner started this incredible chain of events.

- Your partner's body held and nurtured this new life you can now see and touch.

- You have a deep and growing bond with someone you don't really know yet.

Stay with and cherish these moments of amazement. They recharge and re-enthuse you, especially during the more difficult early days and weeks, when you're responding to your baby's wants and needs at all hours.

 Pregnant Pause

Mayo Clinic researchers find that new dads worry about the health of their babies nearly as obsessively as new mothers do. According to the researchers, 58 percent of new fathers admitted having some form of irrational fear or thoughts about their new sons or daughters.

What I'm suggesting here sounds (and may even be) simple. However, simple doesn't always equal easy. To be and feel successful in your fathering, you need constructive attitudes. Unlike most life circumstances, most of your attitudes are within your control. What attitudes help a dad the most?

- **Patience:** Having the endurance, serenity, and strength to stay in the many moments of fatherhood—even if they are sometimes puzzling or frustrating

- **Acceptance:** Understanding and recognizing that there are things you cannot change—such as your child's unique personality—and then finding ways to enjoy those things

- **Faith:** Trusting you and your child can (and will) find ways to handle whatever the present and the future bring

- **Loving detachment:** Loving your child even if you don't always love his behavior

- **Openness:** Being open to learning, new experiences (including new emotions), the ways your child is different than you, and so on

- **Respect for others:** Showing your child you value other people and that it's impossible to gain respect from anyone by disrespecting others

- **Mindfulness:** For instance, if your child throws a tantrum, not responding in kind (what psychologists call a neutral/ empathic response to high stimulus)

- **Discretion:** Knowing when to let loose and be childlike with your child and when to be the grown-up who sets loving limits (even if he doesn't like them)

- **Patience:** Again, being calm and having stamina are good for you and your child

By embracing these constructive attitudes, you not only become a better father, you become a better person. However, like any cause and effect, you have to provide the energy—in other words, continue to practice these attitudes and characteristics. You won't do it perfectly, but that's okay. (Remember Chapter 1, when you read about the value of mistakes?)

Exhibit A: Patience

You may remember from Chapter 4 that your partner's pregnancy is a perfect time to practice the skills and attitudes you'll need as a dad. (You have read the rest of the book, right?) This is now the time to implement what you've learned.

Think about the first (and last) attitude on the preceding list: patience. When your partner was pregnant, you may have had times where nothing you did to calm or comfort her seems to work, which led to you feeling incredibly frustrated. With experience and practice, however, you learned what works best with your partner most of the time (if not every time). This knowledge probably helped reinforce your patience as you rode out the rough patches, because they always ended eventually.

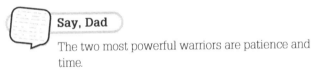

Say, Dad

The two most powerful warriors are patience and time.

—Leo Nikolayevich Tolstoy, author

Your infant will have "impossible" days, too. You may do everything you can to comfort him but still feel like his crying will never stop. At those times, keep the experiences from the pregnancy in mind— you now know that it will end, so you should be able to ride out the more trying times with patience.

On the other hand, it's likely you and your partner had some wonderful moments together during the pregnancy as you contemplated what was happening then and what was ahead. The incredible physical bond your partner experienced with your child then can mirror the mysterious, visceral bond that is now developing between you and your child.

Relish this connection between you and your baby. You'll see unbelievable growth and development in your infant (if you're paying the least bit of attention!). And as his dad, you'll be in touch with the miracle of your baby's life in a way no one else can be. Those are the times when you'll feel like the roles have been reversed, and it's your baby who's giving *you* new life.

You may not feel that heavenly bond all the time; there will still be days you'll feel frustrated, disjointed, and disconnected from your baby. But if you immerse yourself in the good days—and use them to nurture your constructive attitudes—you'll have enough reserves of energy and hope to get you successfully through the bad days … and back into the next good ones.

Creating Your Vision

Men (like most humans) like to be noticed and remembered. Ideally, like other men, you want to be remembered for a long time, motivating you to leave a legacy. The importance of legacy tends to intensify when you have a child or stepchild.

After your child arrives, you may wonder, *What will my child respect and appreciate about me when he's an adult? Will he resent or hate me? How will my child remember me when I'm gone?*

John Badalament, one of today's most innovative and practical fatherhood thinkers and the creator of moderndads.net (he also teaches, makes films, and writes books), encourages men to create a "vision statement" for their fathering. Like your birth plan (see Chapter 10), it's a flexible and adjustable blueprint. Unlike the birth plan, however, a vision statement doesn't prepare you for a single day; instead, it can remain in service for all your days and years of being a dad.

According to John, to make a vision statement, start by imagining that 20 or more years have passed and a documentary filmmaker has come along to interview your child about *you*. You then write down five things you hope your child *would* say about you as a man and a father. Next, write down another five things you hope he *wouldn't* say. These two lists give you materials to build your fathering vision.

Now, starting with the "positive" list, take at least two items to explore. You then write down the following:

- What you're doing *today* to develop a relationship with your child (and others) to facilitate the positive outcome you hope for. (Believe it or not, you're already developing your relationship, even though your baby's a newborn.)

- What you will do *in the future* to develop a relationship with your child (and others) to facilitate this positive outcome.

Next, take the "negative" list and write down the following:

- What you need to stop doing (in your relationship with your child and others).

- What you need to do more of, now and in the future.

John's exercise looks simple and straightforward, but it may feel difficult to complete. That's okay. You're attempting something important—life-changing, in fact—for you and your child. As you flesh out your responses, however, you'll develop a clearer vision of how *you* want to practice the art of fathering.

Say, Dad

Letting your father know how grateful you are is among the greatest gifts a son can give.

—John Badalament, author and speaker on fatherhood

Your responses don't have to be earth shattering. You may look at your words and think, *Well, duh, this is just common sense.* Good for you! However, don't let this diminish the value of your vision statement—or the power of making it concrete and visible in writing.

Your fathering vision statement isn't done yet; it requires two more steps.

First, write down examples of the skills, knowledge, and support you believe you'll need to fulfill your fathering vision. Be specific in all three categories; you can ask for help from some veteran dads (including your own stepdad or dad) and your partner if you feel stumped. Then, organize your work into a simple and specific vision that feels accessible and useable for you.

Finally, share the document with someone trustworthy. You can sign it in that person's presence to signify your commitment to your vision, and then have him or her co-sign as a witness to your pledge.

After it's complete, re-read your fathering vision statement while your child is still an infant, and again regularly over the years to come. Feel free to modify it as you gain more insight and inspiration from experience—and from your child.

The "M" Word

As you read in Chapter 9, marriage brings some legal, financial, and tax benefits to spouses. However, marriage proposals seldom begin with, "Honey, let's tie the knot so we can save $593.41 on next year's tax return." Ideally, you get married because you deeply love your partner, you find the other person interesting, you've learned that you are compatible, and you each want to make a lifelong commitment to your relationship with each other.

At the same time, it's wise to realize that marriage doesn't perfect your relationship; it'll still need nurturing, tinkering, and growth. Marriage also doesn't guarantee the lifelong bit, any more than living together "outside" marriage guarantees that the relationship won't last long.

A growing number of parents do not marry before or after they have children. (Getting married *while* having a child might be tricky, since your partner's concentration is elsewhere.) Nevertheless, marriage questions remain powerful within intimate relationships—and in the larger society.

Marital Benefits

If you follow discussions of principles and practices at fatherhood conferences or in public policy pronouncements, you've heard the term "marriage promotion." Many people in the responsible fatherhood field argue that marriage is vital—if not an essential prerequisite—for successful fathering.

They will cite research showing that married parents are less likely to live in poverty than unmarried parents. The data is accurate, but that doesn't translate into an undisputable truth that marriage prevents poverty.

 Say, Dad

Marriage is a wonderful institution, but who wants to live in an institution?

—Groucho Marx, comedian and actor

By the time you read this, I will have been married for more than 34 years. (Those are consecutive years of marriage, all to the same person.) Having lived (so far) almost two thirds of my life in one, I'm a big fan of marriage.

While I think there's a lot to recommend marriage as a foundation for a stable family, I'm very skeptical of the notion that it's the only foundation. That's because I've witnessed children grow up safely and well in the following family situations:

- Their parents never married.

- Their parents married after they were born.

- Their parents are no longer married.

- Their unmarried parents are no longer a couple.

- One or more of their parents died.

- They have stepparents or the unmarried equivalent.

As you've gleaned from earlier chapters, marriage supplies some significant benefits due to legislation, customs, and cultural attitudes. Unmarried parents will have to invest effort and vigilance to assure the respect and resources that married parents can take for granted. Still, whatever your marital status, your obligation to your children never changes.

Your influence also remains powerful if you live in another home than your child's, you are deployed, your relationship with your partner—or future partner—changes, you are employed or not, and you are in good health or bad. You even influence your child after you die. This is a big part of what makes becoming a father so exciting and challenging. Married or unmarried, you have life-changing obligations to your new child, every one of which is also a wonderful opportunity!

Judgment Calls

On the social front, you'll surely run into people (including relatives) who are less than pleased you had a baby "outside" of marriage. They will include people who think marriage should always come before pregnancy (and intercourse), or people who think it's wrong for homosexual couples or single people to give birth or adopt. When dealing with these attitudes, be open, honest, and accepting and roll with the punches.

 Pregnant Pause

Your commitment to your child and your partner are far more important than a relative's disapproving comments. Don't let people's opinions derail you from staying on track to be deeply involved in your child's life.

For example, I adored my grandfather and always craved his approval, so it hurt when he told me how disappointed he was my partner and I got pregnant several months before we were married. But being the wise man he was, he didn't belabor the point (since he knew this wouldn't stop the birth), and he didn't stop showing his love. He only lived a few years longer, but he said that one of the happiest days of his life was our visit when our twins were 9 months old. He joyfully sat his creaky, 80-something body down on the floor so he could gurgle, chatter, and laugh with his first two great-grandchildren.

His delight that day erased any hurt and anxiety I'd felt. After all, a happy great-grandfather was far more important for my kids than whether my feelings were bruised the year before.

So sure, a relative's reaction may hurt for a short time. But if everyone acts like an adult, the hurt will soon be forgotten in the excitement of your beautiful baby.

If some people choose not to act like adults, well, there's nothing you can do to change them, so don't try. You're far better off putting that energy into raising your kid well, so that when he becomes an adult, *he'll* act like one.

Guarding Against Gatekeeping

This section is written specifically for *both* you and your partner to read. Share it with other relatives, too, if you'd like—however, make sure your partner reads it.

Back in the first chapter, I talked about how girls generally get more training and practice at childrearing than boys do. Therefore, people tend to think of females as more suited to the job of raising kids, and they sometimes are.

However, this is a cultural phenomenon; men and women aren't "hard-wired" to have more or less parenting capacity. Through both subtle and blatant means, our culture effectively makes moms defend the domain of childhood.

Even in families fully committed to equal parenting, the mother often becomes the gatekeeper of childrearing, keeping some things in and other things out. For example, the mother usually does the feeding, schedules the sitter, instructs the father and babysitter on the proper way to change diapers, and is the one who gets the baby when he won't stop crying. Meanwhile, the father defers and stays "outside" the center of childrearing because that's what he's sup-posed to do. He's no expert—and who isn't tempted to avoid a dirty diaper?

 Say, Dad

When you make the sacrifice in marriage, you're sacrificing not to each other but to unity in a relationship.

—Joseph Campbell, writer

Let me be absolutely clear: mothers and fathers don't fall into gate-keeping patterns in order to win some sort of power struggle, get back at each other, or because one loves the children more than the other. Gatekeeping happens because people grew up learning to arbitrarily divide parenting responsibilities by gender. Malevolence has nothing to do with it. Most of the time, this setup is done unconsciously and with the best intentions. It may even seem like the best arrangement.

But a "mother-knows-best" model only looks logical if you accept the screwy cultural notion that childrearing is "women's work" while bread-winning is "men's work." Of course, such beliefs leave you out, make more work for your partner, and leave everyone in the family with father hunger.

Blue and Pink Chores

Centuries ago when I was a kid, I mowed the lawn and emptied the garbage—traditional boy chores. One night my sister asked why my chores only needed doing one day a week, while she had to cook or wash clothes and dishes every day. My mom replied, "Joe will learn to clean and cook in the Army." I never knew my mother could be so sexist! Besides, she never wanted me to go into the Army. Fortunately, my sister didn't hold this against me. Years later, she and her husband bought us two months' worth of diaper ser-vice when our kids were born, perhaps the most useful gift I've ever received!

Outdated attitudes about dividing things up by "women's work" and "men's work" simply don't cut the mustard if you want to be a truly involved dad getting the most out of fathering. With the one exception of breastfeeding, you're capable of doing anything and everything parental. So take on an equal (if not a bit more than equal) load of everything else that must be done.

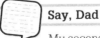 **Say, Dad**

My second favorite household chore is ironing. My first is hitting my head on the top bunk bed until I faint.

—Erma Bombeck, newspaper reporter and humorist

The two of you are putting your primary energies into the baby himself, as you should. But meals still need to be cooked, clothes washed, dishes done, and floors vacuumed. You're all better off if both of you share the most essential tasks around the house.

My friend Chris recommends, "Do half the work, all the time, 24 hours a day, 7 days a week, 52 weeks a year. Always be a parent, never be a babysitter." In practical execution, this approach requires figuring out with your partner what this means. Suppose you hate doing laundry and she hates cleaning the bathroom and mopping floors. So she does most of the laundry and you clean the bathroom and mop the floors. When it comes to infant care, the division of labor is fairly straightforward:

- Change (at least) half the diapers.

- Give half the baths.

- Do (at least) half the feedings—if the baby isn't breastfeeding, of course.

- Do half the nighttime rocking chair and baby walking duty.

If your parents were like mine and didn't make you do inside-the-house chores, you may wish you had a guide to doing laundry. My publisher can't justify such a tome, since it'd be less than 10 pages long. So instead, read the washing machine manual and the detergent bottle label; they're written for the most inexperienced launderers.

In addition, switch to easily washed and dried clothes. Permanent-press shirts are very attractive after a few weeks with an infant; why iron when you could be playing with the baby? Even if you run one of your partner's delicate sweaters through the dryer, remember that sweaters can be replaced—time with your child can't.

And even if you've never cooked before, you are smart enough to follow a recipe and make some simple, nutritious meals.

For goodness sake, don't get hung up believing that cooking and cleaning are unmanly. Cooking, cleaning, burping, changing diapers, earning money, comforting tears—it's all parents' work. Only a fool divvies up those necessary tasks by arbitrary (and silly) concepts of gender roles. Think about it; would you tell a U.S. Marine peeling potatoes in the mess or cleaning out a field latrine that he isn't a real man?

Different Isn't Dumb

Moms and dads do things differently. In fact, regardless of gender, any two parents will do things differently because they're two different people. (The same goes for stepparents, grandparents, cousins, and any other caregivers.) Kids benefit from the difference, so you and your partner have to make sure your child is exposed to both parenting styles.

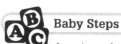 **Baby Steps**

A review of empirical research in the National Council of Family Relations journal shows there are more similarities than differences between how dads and moms interact with infants. In reality, you and your partner have similar childrearing desires, goals, and challenges. Put energy into what you have in common, learn from one another, and cheer each other on.

To calm a crying infant, you may sit with perfect quiet in a rocking chair, slowly easing him to sleep. To calm that same crying infant, your partner may walk the floor, jabber nonsense, and bounce him on her knee until he tires and goes to sleep.

One way isn't better, worse, smarter, or dumber than the other, since both methods got the baby to stop crying and go to sleep. Even better, the baby is learning two important things:

- There's more than one way to bond with and be nurtured by an adult who cares for him.

- There's more than one way he can (eventually) calm and relax himself.

Parenting research indicates that a father is more likely to carry an infant so he's facing away from him, while a mother is more likely to carry the baby facing toward her. Which one is better?

That's precisely the wrong question. Parenting is not a competition, and your baby is not a football. Seductive as it may be to fall into patterns of scorekeeping—"I do (fill in the blank) better/more often than my partner does"—keeping score harms your child. And it's lousy for your relationship with each other.

In addition, people tend to judge or rank different baby-care strategies not based on whether they work in the end, but rather on how closely they mirror an artificially "gendered" method, which many probably grew up thinking was the "right" one.

Your baby needs *both* perspectives. It's good for him to explore the world, and it's good for him to know his family intimately. It doesn't matter which parent provides which—and there's every reason for both you and your partner to provide a little bit of each.

The key is to remember that an infant has more than one parent for very good reasons. Don't let yourself or your partner be locked out, because that's not good for your child.

Opening the Gate

You both need to be aware of the gates that may shut out fully shared parenting. The most obvious one during your baby's first year is breastfeeding. Of course, no matter how hard you try, you can't share breastfeeding "equally." So does that mean "extra points" for your partner? Well, yes and no.

Yes, because you should admire and respect breastfeeding as a major, time-consuming commitment which brings incredible benefit to your baby. No, because assigning "points" (even unconsciously) sets a hard-to-break pattern of comparing the value of parental contribution X with the value of parental contribution Y.

Follow that path, and you're soon in binding thickets of tension of who gets to assign and weigh "value" and pointless scorekeeping ... which inevitably leads to the toxic swamp of resentment.

Instead, think "outside the gate" to develop an ethos of shared parenting. After all, there are even ways to share with breastfeeding (see Chapter 12)!

 Say, Dad

It is not a lack of love, but a lack of friendship that makes unhappy marriages.

—Friedrich Nietzsche, philosopher

For over 20 years, I've discussed and wrestled with the gatekeeping dynamic with parents in North America and overseas. I see no point in finding someone to "blame" for gatekeeping. Instead, I've interviewed and corresponded with parents to come up with ideas for shifting out of the habit.

Here's what I've learned:

- Both men and women are complicit in continuing this deeply entrenched cultural habit. That means men and women also must share the work of replacing gatekeeping with a better parenting framework.

- While learning (like reading this book) is necessary for good fathering, it is not itself sufficient. A dad-to-be has to act on what he learns in this book, from other parents, and from himself. That's a man's first step.

- It's great for your pregnant partner (or any other relatives) to read about and reflect on gatekeeping. However, a mom-to-be also has to act on her insights, challenging internalized ideas and assumptions about the parenting capacity of women and men. She must act in ways that expect, demand, and support the father's inclusion, rather than reinforce patterns of leaving him on the outside looking in.

If this sounds good in theory, how does it work in practice? Here are some practical ideas—most of them from veteran mothers:

- If your baby *is not* breastfeeding, you should feed him just as often as your partner does.

- If your baby *is* breastfeeding, you should hold him, play with him, and put him to sleep just as often as your partner does (or even a little bit more).

- When you're holding your baby and he won't stop crying, you should take the time and space to figure out your own solution. The same goes for your partner.

- Advise and encourage each other; don't hover.

- Think before you "rescue." You both have plenty to learn about this child. Your child will teach you every day how many important lessons come from mistakes (see Chapter 1). So, don't keep each other from your mistakes. (A good attitude to have with your child, too, when he's older.)

Remember, the two of you may have different ways of feeding, burping, changing, and comforting your baby. You may also have different ways of playing with him or getting him to drop off to sleep.

This is a good thing!

So look out for gatekeeping and talk openly when either of you spot it (in each other, relatives, or friends). Don't fall into blaming; gatekeeping doesn't happen unless you both let it happen.

Do your best to expect and encourage each other to fully share the obligations, opportunities, and joys of raising your children together.

Okay, your partner doesn't have to read anymore. But if she does, make sure she talks about it with you!

Caring for a Child with Birth Defects

Raising a child with chronic physical or intellectual challenges will test you on many levels. There will be strains on your psyche, your marriage, other family relationships, your place in society, and the well-being of your new baby.

Over the years, you will face barriers as concrete as a set of stairs and as ephemeral as social prejudice against people with "disabilities." You will face mundane challenges like bathing your child, and lifelong challenges like how to provide for him when you're gone.

The Language of "Defects"

In the United States, approximately 150,000 babies are born each year with a serious condition that falls under the general term of "birth defect." Of course, there is logic in referring to something like spina bifida or Down syndrome as a birth defect. But the language of "defect" or "disability" has serious shortcomings.

 Pregnant Pause

A child with Down syndrome doesn't think of himself as a walking birth defect. He thinks of himself as a son, grandson, nephew, friend, student—as a kid. That's how his parents—and the rest of us—should see him, too.

After all, every one of us has something that could be described as a defect. I've never been able to hit (or throw) a curveball and I'm right-handed. If the standard is being a National League southpaw pitcher, I have some serious birth defects. This may seem like a silly example, but the point is that humans have differing abilities. That means we all have various disabilities, too. Does this matter?

Most people don't think of themselves as having "disabilities," even though their own abilities will change gradually (due to age) or suddenly (due to disease, accident, and so on). Instead, if you think about it at all, you think of yourself as a person who needs glasses to read or drive, not as a semi-blind man.

Nevertheless, we might tend to see children in the special education class as "retarded," damaged, and pitiable burdens on society—rather than as kids who have, among other things (like legs and fingers), Down syndrome.

Whether people's language puts the kid before or after his birth defect says a lot about whether you as a parent put your kid before or after his birth defect. Your words also frame how you value your child—and the adult he'll become. Just remember, the person belongs first and the disability second.

Medical and Legal Issues

Author and advocate Janet Morel says that, as parents of a child with special needs, "You will have to become like the mother bear protecting her young." You will need to immediately advocate for your child, making sure he gets what he needs and deserves: good medical care, education, adaptive tools like wheelchairs, a safe and loving group home or other facility, and so on.

You also have to think about money. A 2005 national U.S. study reported that 40 percent of families of children with special health-care needs experience a financial burden due to their child's condition (see ncbi.nlm.nih.gov/pmc/articles/PMC1802121/). You should immediately address your financial situation, your insurance, and your will so your child can be properly cared for should something happen to you. The Pacer Center, which advocates for children with disabilities, has a good general publication on financial issues for parents at pacer.org/publications/possibilities. Your child may be eligible for assistance through SSI, or Social Security disability (see socialsecuritydisability.tv/blog/what-different-birth-defects-qualify-for-social-security-disability).

In addition, be sure to talk openly and often with your partner and your extended families about what you both want for your child down the road.

Fortunately, there are organizations, support groups, and professionals who can help you advocate effectively and maintain your energy. The National Institute of Child Health and Human Development (nichd.nih.gov/health/topics/birthdefects/resources/Pages/patients.aspx), The Arc of the United States (thearc.org), and the National Dissemination Center for Children with Disabilities (http://nichcy.org/) are good places to start looking for links to these resources.

While dealing with these important medical and legal matters, you may also have to advocate getting the extended family support, love, and affection that you, your partner, and your child deserve. So get ready to be brave, persistent, and insistent.

Responding to and Resisting Stereotypes

You're liable to experience a mixture of intense emotions if you have a child with unexpected but chronic issues. Like every new father, you're thrilled to see him, hold him, and begin bonding with this unique person you helped create.

At the same time, you may feel sadness, fear, and anxiety about his future. You may worry about his health, life expectancy, education and career prospects, how you will handle all the responsibility, and where you'll find the support and money you'll need. You may feel angry and resentful toward the medical community, God, or whoever else you think is responsible for his condition—you may even be angry at yourself.

 Attention, Please

Anger, anxiety, and sadness are all normal reactions. They don't mean you don't or can't love your new child, or that you're not qualified to raise him.

It's natural to ask, "Why him?" or "Why me?" However, those questions are seldom (if ever) useful. There may be no answers, and you can't know exactly what happened. "This agonizes some parents," according to psychologist Kitty Westin, whose adult son has needed specialized care from birth. "I have talked with parents who spend their energy and much of their life looking for an answer … but, don't blame your partner or yourself. This only creates discord, fuels anger, causes sadness and distracts from the important work—and joy—of loving your child for who she or he is."

You can love your child and still feel afraid or sad. Just realize that it doesn't help to ask "*Why* us?" Instead, ask, "*How* can we respond to our child and our circumstances?" You can find the support you need to raise your child successfully if you have the courage, openness, and determination to seek it.

For example, you may feel grief while anticipating your child will never ride a bike or play catch with you. However, that thought process is flawed. Children and adults with disabilities *do* learn to ride bikes, play catch, swim, shoot golf, and engage in other activities. They may use different methods, venues, support, and equipment to participate, but they do participate—often with their family members.

Therefore, there's no reason to perceive these pursuits and hobbies as "less than" the way you play a game. For proof, watch some wheelchair basketball. Those athletes are not "confined to a wheelchair." Wheelchairs don't limit their basketball ability. Instead, these men and women use the chairs to flaunt their moves!

Of course, improved perceptions alone can't prevent your parenting road from giving bumps and bruises to you, your partner, and your child. Some of these will be the same as other parents' experience, and some will be different. Resenting or bemoaning the difference won't get you where you need to go.

Writer and disabled activist Bill Trzeciak recommends, "As best you can, just keep your eyes on the road and steer around the potholes as you spot them. Watch for oncoming traffic to avoid (like people who don't yet get it) and you and your family should come out okay."

And to help you get past the expectations of yourself and others for raising a "normal" child, Bill suggests considering something you may never have perceived before: Start by asking how much of your sorrow or anxiety grows from deeply rooted cultural beliefs and expectations about what's "normal."

Advocates for disability rights argue that "disability" itself is an artificial social construct that ignores and denies the diversity of human characteristics. Children and adults with chronic conditions have been in (if not always full members of) our communities and families for millennia. Because these people diverge from our expectations of "normal," you may feel afraid, sad, and sometimes ashamed—a poisonous posture for parents.

How can you resist the corrosive feelings and responses to your child's condition? As some anonymous sage once said, "Look for what you have in common with others, rather than how you are different."

For example, a child with chronic conditions will certainly demand more time, energy, and resources than you expected. Then again, a "perfectly healthy" baby will also demand more time, energy, and resources than you expected (trust me). So look for support from other parents and community resources—just like every parent should.

Recognize that fathers of children with and without "disabilities" can (and do) feel the deep joys and satisfaction of raising their kids. And that's precisely what your child needs most.

A Final Word

You read this book to help stake a central role in the pregnancy you and your partner are sharing. Ideally, you also want to be a key player on the first day of your child's life.

You've demonstrated intense attention and commitment to this pregnancy and childbirth. You're willing to go to classes, protect and nurture your partner, make sacrifices, and go joyously through the chaotic miracle of labor and delivery.

Your next challenge is to take this same intensity into every day of your new baby's childhood. Your child needs your deep commitment and involvement. If you have a boy, he needs you to show him how to hug, bake cookies, snowshoe, and be someone who respects loved ones. If you have a girl, she needs you to show her how to drive a nail, jump off the high dive, tie a lure … and be someone who respects loved ones.

You'll cherish the times you teach your child important skills, shining with pride when those skills are mastered. But the heart of fathering is nurturing the psychological, emotional, and spiritual connection between you and your child.

For pioneering fathering author Will Glennon, a dad's biggest challenge isn't mastering the "proper" way to change a diaper or teach your kid to read—it's to set aside obsolete attitudes about a father's role and to begin fathering from the heart.

Fathering is too good an experience for you or your child to miss. So, please, show up for it every day. You'll be amazed before you're halfway through.

Those of us who already have children welcome you into the fraternity of fathers. We're honored to have you in our fellowship. May you relish your membership every day.

The Least You Need to Know

- Practicing strong, positive attitudes will enrich your fathering and make you a good role model to your child.

- You can create your own vision statement for the art of being a dad, which you can then refer to as your child grows.

- Despite what "marriage promotion" advocates say, you can be a good father to your child even if you aren't married to your partner.

- Moving beyond gatekeeping and other traditional gender roles takes work, but it's worth the effort.

- Taking care of a special-needs child involves advocating for your child and challenging the notion of what's "normal."

Index

Symbols

A

B

D

J–K

L

Printed in Great Britain
by Amazon